Spirits Captured
in Stone

Spirits Captured in Stone

Shamanism and Traditional Medicine Among the Taman of Borneo

Jay H. Bernstein

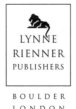

LYNNE
RIENNER
PUBLISHERS

BOULDER
LONDON

Published in the United States of America in 1997 by
Lynne Rienner Publishers, Inc.
1800 30th Street, Boulder, Colorado 80301

and in the United Kingdom by
Lynne Rienner Publishers, Inc.
3 Henrietta Street, Covent Garden, London WC2E 8LU

Library of Congress Cataloging-in-Publication Data
Bernstein, Jay H., 1959–
    Spirits captured in stone : shamanism and traditional medicine
    among the Taman of Borneo / Jay H. Bernstein.
    Includes bibliographical references and index.
    ISBN 1-55587-691-9 (hc : alk. paper)
    ISBN 1-55587-692-7 (pbk. : alk. paper)
    1. Taman (Bornean people)—Religion.   2. Taman (Bornean people)—
    Medicine.   3. Taman (Bornean people)—Rites and ceremonies.
    4. Traditional medicine—Borneo.   5. Shamanism—Borneo.   6. Borneo—
    Social life and customs.   I. Title.
    DS646.32.T35B47   1996
    299'.92—dc20   96-43233
                                                                          CIP

British Cataloguing in Publication Data
A Cataloguing in Publication record for this book
is available from the British Library.

Printed and bound in the United States of America

        The paper used in this publication meets the requirements
   ∞ of the American National Standard for Permanence of
        Paper for Printed Library Materials Z39.48-1984-1984.

    5 4 3 2 1

To my parents, and to the memory of Kenneth W. Payne

Contents

Preface

Fieldwork is culturally subversive. It temporarily detaches one from one's own way of thinking and doing, yet it never entirely connects to an alternate one. It fosters one's imagination about both. The better one empathizes, the better one does ethnography, yet full absorption and empathy within another world would inhibit social insight. For these reasons, one could argue that anthropology . . . is a tragic discipline in that it goes far to isolate and alienate its practitioners from full conviction in their own mode of thinking and doing.
—*T. O. Beidelman* (1993, p. 214)

As a graduate student wanting to master the literature on Southeast Asian ethnography and hoping someday to make an original contribution to anthropology, I came across two books written in the 1950s by W. R. Geddes on the Land Dayak people (now known as Bidayuh), who inhabit an area in western Borneo including parts of both Sarawak (Malaysia) and West Kalimantan (Indonesia). I was intrigued by these books and eventually resolved that I would undertake a full-scale ethnographic study of the Bidayuh, concentrating on questions of medical knowledge and rationality and using the perspectives of cognitive anthropology, the sociology of knowledge, and the situational analysis of case histories. Shamanism was mentioned only in passing in my proposal, and I fully expected to concentrate on folk medicines made from natural materials. I make no apology that this book, finished many years later, takes a different outlook from the one I originally proposed. All experienced anthropologists know that anything they write in their proposals turns out, one way or another, to be unworkable, uninteresting, or wrong by the time they get to the field. Furthermore, anthropology itself has moved ahead since 1983. Although much of this is a matter of styling, fads, and new words for old ideas, there is more to it than that. Theoretical approaches concerning many issues such as gender, material culture, performance, medical aesthetics, medical discourse, and embodiment have matured greatly in this time, and I have tried to relate my findings to some of these developments. At the same time, I recognize that the important and enduring questions of belief, knowledge, and reality are still with us in social and medical anthropology, and that it is better to confront these issues than to get carried away by fads.

By the time I wrote my research proposal, I had ascertained that Sarawak was closed to foreign researchers, so I proposed to do a study of the Bidayuh in West Kalimantan. In September 1984, after taking an advanced course in the Indonesian language at Satya Wacana Christian University in Java, I traveled throughout most of West Kalimantan in search of a suitable locale for a project on cognitive processes and knowledge domains in traditional medicine. I was unable to visit any Bidayuh settlements, but a minister from West Kalimantan who was finishing his thesis on the Taman for a degree in theology from Satya Wacana and who was married to a Taman woman arranged to take me to some Taman villages. During these brief visits, my interest in these people was stimulated both by their traditional village life and by what I was learning about their folk healers, so I settled on doing my work among the Taman. The main fieldwork was carried out from late 1985 to early 1987 and from mid-1987 to early 1988. This book's ethnographic present corresponds to those periods of time.

My research was funded by an International Doctoral Research Fellowship from the Social Science Research Council with the American Council of Learned Societies and an Individual National Research Service Award from the National Institute of Mental Health. I gratefully acknowledge the financial support of these organizations and from the Graduate Division of the University of California, Berkeley, and the Luce Foundation. I was sponsored by the Bureau of International Relations of the Indonesian Institute of Sciences (Lembaga Ilmu Pengetahuan Indonesia), through the Center for Environmental Studies (Pusat Penelitian Lingkungan Hidup) of Gadjah Mada National University. I thank the center's director, Sugeng Martopo, and its secretary, Djalal Tandjung, for their backing. Michael Dove was especially instrumental in helping me realize my goal of carrying out this study, and his moral support over the years since then has been a sustaining force. I also thank the faculty of Tanjungpura National University for their help and advice.

I am deeply indebted to all my informants, who must remain anonymous. (I have replaced all personal names with pseudonyms in the text.) However, it would be ungracious of me not to thank by name my fine hosts, F. Gunding and family in Sibau Hilir and M. Layang and family in Tanjung Lasa. I also thank the Reverend A. Iking and his family in Putussibau for their hospitality, which made my continued research possible. His church, the Gereja Kalimantan Evangelis, facilitated my work in countless ways. Cornelius Kimha in Putussibau and Dharsono in Pontianak were true friends through thick and thin, when I was beset by desperate problems in the field. The favors and cheerful correspondence of John McVey and David

Rosenthal helped me preserve my affairs at home as well as my sanity during that time.

I am grateful to the friends, teachers, and colleagues who read early versions of the text and whose critiques and suggestions for revision helped me improve it: James N. Anderson, Burton Benedict, Jeanne L. Bergman, Donald E. Brown, George A. De Vos, Marco Jacquemet, Ondina F. Leal, Lyn Lowry, Mary Porter, Lesley Sharp, Amin Sweeney, and Robert L. Winzeler. I thank the University of Kent at Canterbury for its institutional support and especially Roy Ellen for all he has done for me. I am also indebted to Yvette Mead for her assistance with a translation and to Nicole Bourque, whose brainstorms led to the book's title.

An earlier debt is to the late Kenneth W. Payne, who became my mentor in 1978 and was my closest friend for the next ten years. To a great extent he set my work in a certain direction, and his loyal backing from the beginning helped make it possible for me to pursue a career in anthropology.

I am forever indebted to my parents, Joseph and Flora Bernstein, for their enduring love, support, patience, and faith in me when the chips were down. Finally, I acknowledge my gratitude to Budi Bernstein, Jordan Bernstein, Jason Bernstein, and Bruce Bernstein.

Jay H. Bernstein

Note on Transcription

Taman pronunciation is similar to that of the Indonesian language, which has been described by Echols and Shadily (1989: xiv–xvii), and with a few exceptions, it may be adequately transcribed using standard Indonesian orthography. These exceptions are the use in Taman of elongated /a/, /i/, /l/, and /o/ sounds, represented here by /aa/, /ii/, /ll/, and /oo/, and the glottal stop, represented by /'/. With these exceptions, I have transcribed Taman speech as I would Indonesian.

The major drawback of using conventional Indonesian transcription is that it does not account for the variety of pronunciations of /e/. Sometimes it is ɛ, as in *bed*. (This pronunciation is used in the word *balien*.) Other times it is ∂, like the first *e* in *decide*. Unlike the pronunciation of the word prefixes /me-/ and /meng-/ in the Indonesian language, the /e/ in these prefixes is intermediate between /∂/ and /a/. At the end of a word it is E, as in *say*.

Barring these irregularities, the rest of Taman orthography is straightforward.

Vowels

/i/ high, front, unrounded, close; like *ee* as in *feel* but shorter
/a/ low, central, unrounded, open; like *o* in *rock*
/o/ mid, back, rounded, open; like *o* in *fold*
/u/ high, back, rounded, close; like *oo* in *tool*

Consonants

/b/ voiced labial stop, like *b* in *bar*
/c/ alveopalatal fricative, like *ch* in *charge*
/d/ voiced alveolar stop, like *d* in *David*
/g/ voiced velar stop, like *g* in *girl*
/h/ voiceless glottal fricative, like *h* in *how*

/j/ voiced alveopalatal fricative, like *j* in *jump*
/k/ voiceless velar stop, like *c* in *car,* but without puff of air
/l/ voiced alveolar lateral, like *l* in *lemon*
/m/ voiced labial nasal, like *m* in *mountain*
/n/ voiced alveolar nasal, like *n* in *name*
/ng/ voiced velar nasal, like *ng* in *sing*
/ny/ voiced palatal nasal, like *ny* in *canyon*
/p/ voiceless labial stop, like *p* in *lip,* but without puff of air
/r/ voiced velar trill, like *r* in *very British.* N.B. Malay pronunciation is
     trilled as in French *rêve.*
/s/ voiceless alveolar fricative, like *s* in *send*
/t/ voiceless alveolar stop, like *t* in *let,* but without puff of air
/w/ voiced labial semivowel, like *w* in *wow*
/y/ voiced palatal semivowel, like *y* in *yell*

In Taman as in Indonesian, the accent usually falls on the penultimate syllable. Thus, the word *menyarung* is pronounced me-NYA-rung. However, the word *balien* is pronounced with stress on the final syllable or shared between the first and the last syllable.

1

Introduction

The Taman Balien

This book examines the healing practices of the Taman, an ethnic group of 4,500 people living in the interior of Indonesian Borneo. In particular, it focuses on the objects, practices, and activities of certain shamanistic healers called *balien* and the concepts underlying this institutionalized folk-medical occupation. The Taman believe that many illnesses—both major and minor—originate in the work of spirits. Baliens can treat only those illnesses; however, treatment by a balien may be all that is available to the ailing person without leaving the Taman village.

The balien treats illnesses presumed to have been caused by spirits that have attacked or disturbed a person's soul. In some cases, the soul is thought to have left the person's body and been taken away by a spirit. The balien is able to feel disease-objects and remove them from the body; to see, hear, and catch spirits; and to locate, capture, and replace lost souls. The use of medicines in balien treatments is secondary to the use of special healing stones, which occupy a central role in all the balien's techniques. These stones are considered by the Taman to have magical powers and to be of miraculous origin, and the crux of the balien system lies in their mystery.

The balien's repertoire consists of seven ceremonies, ranked in order of their level of advancement. No one but a balien may perform any of these ceremonies. The balien is compensated for his or her work but does not subsist on payments. Outside the performance of these ceremonies, the balien is not differentiated from any other Taman adult and has no particular advantages or disadvantages.

Most remarkable about the balien system is that the highest of the balien's ceremonies is the inauguration of a patient as a balien. The predisposing condition of the balien is not caring for the sick but rather suffering illness: The balien has been transformed from a sick person and the subject of treatment into a healer. From the Taman point of view, the person initiat-

ed as a balien has been transformed not so much in social status as in metaphysical status because of his or her intimacy with the spirit realm, indicated by the ability to see, hear, talk to, and interact with spirits.

The Taman believe that baliens have an involuntary vocation or destiny
for entering this special healing role. They are believed to have been afflicted by a dangerous illness, not curable through conventional (nonbalien)
means, as a result of spirit seduction. Bodily ailments suffered before initiation are reinterpreted as "disturbance" from a spirit who has singled the
person out for victimization. Visions, dreams, preoccupations, and delusions
are indications that the person has been charmed or seduced sexually by one
or more spirits. In treating this illness, a ceremony is held in which a minimum of two baliens invite the various spirits from the surrounding area to
descend and then "catch" them by tapping them with leaves, thereby turning
them into stones. Events following this ceremony, such as the return of the
illness, determine whether the person must be initiated as a balien. The
balien's initiation repeats the preceding ceremony on a grander scale, producing more stones from the concrescence of wild spirits. The stones collected in both ceremonies are given to the novice balien, who uses them in
treating illnesses.

While the balien institution is unique to the Taman in its particular
details, it is also a specific instance of a more widespread phenomenon,
shamanism. In the following sections, I shall describe the state of knowledge
about shamanism in general and the various theories and debates about its
meaning and nature that form the context of a detailed study of the balien
and Taman traditional healing.

Shamanism in General

Definitions of shamanism have been much disputed. The term is most commonly applied to symbolic or magical healing and is related to the idea that
illness is caused by spirits or harm to the soul. By this definition, a shaman
is a healer who effects cures through the flight of the soul and contact with
spirits. Dissent arises because the terms "shamanism" and "shaman" are
sometimes applied to matters other than the cure of illness. The keys to the
definition of shamanism are soul flight and the use of spirit-helpers, who
give the shaman his or her powers. (A shaman may be a man or a woman,
or, in rare instances, a boy or a girl.) However, the shaman's body is not
taken over involuntarily by the spirit-helper; instead, the shaman controls
the contact with the spirit-helper.

The work of the shaman is conducted in a frame of mind that the histo-
rian of religions Mircea Eliade (1964) calls "ecstasy." This term has generally been replaced in the more recent literature by "altered states of consciousness," which subsumes "trance," "spirit possession," and "dissociation" (see Bourguignon 1965; Atkinson 1992). For Eliade, the particular

technique of ecstasy in which the shaman "specializes" is "a trance in which his soul is believed to leave his body and ascend to the sky or descend to the lower world" (Eliade 1964: 5). I. M. Lewis's (1986: 86) observation that shamans can master (or fight) spirits "in this world," as well as in worlds above or below the one in which humans ordinarily live, is pertinent to the Taman case. Whether or not the shaman's soul travels to a world located on a different plane of reality, it is experienced by leaving the body and meeting spirits.

A further point in the definition of shamanism, emphasized by Åke Hultkrantz (1978: 33–38), is that the shaman labors as an intermediary between spirits and humans, on behalf of a human interest.

The word "shaman" itself is derived from Tungus, a Siberian language. As Eliade (1964: 4) says, "shamanism in the strict sense" is pre-eminently a Siberian and Central Asian phenomenon; however, it has spread around the world. The universal importance of animal spirits in shamanism strongly indicates a link with a hunting adaptation (Hultkrantz 1978), and this fact suggests that shamanism played a great part in the evolution of religion, particularly cosmology (see Riches 1994; La Barre 1972).

The widespread prevalence of shamanism among traditional peoples on six continents has enabled this phenomenon to be studied comparatively in both anthropology (Lewis 1971; Winkelman 1992) and the history of religions (Eliade 1964; Hultkrantz 1978). The anthropologist Jane Atkinson (1992) has recently summed up the literature in her essay "Shamanisms Today." As the title suggests, it may be misleading to universalize about shamanism. Shamanism is associated with several distinct functions, not all of which are present in every instance of shamanism. For example, Hultkrantz (1978: 35–37) identifies five main tasks of the shaman that are associated with various roles: doctor, diviner, psychopomp, hunting magician, and sacrificial priest. This complexity of the shaman's role may be attributed to the fact that the shaman is the sole magicoreligious practitioner in simple band societies and as a result must wear several hats.

Approaches to Shamanism in Anthropology

Confusion about shamanism has resulted from the fact that some practices have wrongly been identified as shamanic. Even discounting these errors, there are many kinds of shamans. Anthropologists who study shamanism within a specific setting often give it a particular slant; in so doing, they are perhaps being influenced by their theoretical presuppositions and attitudes. For example, a number of anthropologists who have studied shamanism— such as Dale Valory (1970), who examined the Yurok Indians of California, and Vinson Sutlive (1992), who observed the Iban of the Sibu district in Sarawak—have stressed the psychological deviance of the shaman. In his account of Iban shamanism in the Saribas area, however, Robert Barrett

(1993) emphasizes dramatic performance, following the work of Bruce Kapferer (1991), an anthropologist who studied exorcism and spirit possession in Sri Lanka. Jane Atkinson not only emphasizes the importance of dramatic performance in her study of shamanism among the Wana on the Indonesian island of Sulawesi (Atkinson 1987) but views the institution of shamanism as an instrument of political authority (Atkinson 1989). Anna Tsing, in her book on the Meratus of South Kalimantan, follows an approach to shamanism similar to Atkinson's, stating that

> shamanic spirituality is a key site for the negotiation of Meratus politics. Shamanism forms an important marker of authority within Meratus communities. Shamans distinguish themselves as people worth listening to. They understand power—whether the violence of the military, the ritual of administration, or the magic of religion. They combine authoritative knowledge, articulateness, and the ability to draw an audience; they are thus leaders. (Tsing 1993: 230–231)

In Tsing's (1987) early account of a Meratus Dayak woman shaman, Uma Adang, the status or role of shaman provides a legitimizing soapbox for a creative and eccentric prophet. Tsing's theoretical perspective on Meratus shamanism has since changed drastically. In a subsequent study she describes the same shaman as epitomizing "the postmodernism of marginality" (Tsing 1993: 254). Another such woman is likened to "a structuralist critic," or perhaps a "poststructuralist," since she "deconstructs the taken-for-granted grounds of shamanic representation" and "exposes the gender biases of its excesses and its marginalia" (Tsing 1993: 240). The characterization of Meratus shamans as postmodernist, poststructuralist, and postfeminist is perplexing, but the notion that shamans, especially female shamans, are critics of society is a standard, if partial, explanation for shamanism.

This idea has been developed most notably by I. M. Lewis (1971), with a view toward explaining the social makeup of participants in shamanism and spirit possession. (His discussion of practices conducted mainly or exclusively by women is pertinent to the case at hand, since about 90 percent of Taman baliens are women.) Lewis argues that beneath their apparent concern with disease and its treatment, women's possession cults actually function as "thinly disguised protest movements directed against the dominant sex, [and] thus play a significant part in the sex-war in traditional societies and cultures where women lack more obvious and direct means for forwarding their aims" (Lewis 1971: 31). According to Lewis, shamanism and spirit possession are oblique but deliberate strategies that may be used to express dissatisfaction with social norms that denigrate women. Through possession or membership in a shamanistic group, a woman can ventilate a grudge against a particular man and gain respect, economic security, or luxury goods she might not otherwise acquire. Women's possession cults are characteristic of rigidly patriarchal societies, in which women are subordinated to men, but they are part of the larger phenomenon of cults focusing on the downtrodden strata of society. In societies in which women are not thought of or treated as inferior to men, women do not dominate these cults, and men, especially those who are subordinate or marginal, take part to the same extent as women. Thus, the focus of possession cults may shift over time.

Lewis's hypothesis cannot explain the balien complex with its predominantly female composition. Like traditional Southeast Asian society in general, Taman society is relatively egalitarian with regard to women's status. Baliens treat patients of both sexes, and men as well as women may be treated for illnesses identical to the balien's predisposing illness. Both men and women resist becoming baliens, and men's illnesses are most often resolved before it becomes necessary for them to proceed to the level of initiation. Baliens are mainly healers for the community, and with the exception of an apparently obsolescent ceremony to remove the souls of the dead, they have no broader powers of religious leadership. The spirits causing illness that are used in shamanism are not worshiped in any way, nor are baliens their devotees. Rather, the spirits are, in Lewis's terms, amoral nature spirits, peripheral to the system of morality. Baliens gain little in material terms from their activities; they are neither revered nor despised; and they do little to suggest that they take pleasure in their work. Rather than consciously using illness to attain a more comfortable or powerful lot in life, those who become baliens give the impression of passively accepting their fate. For this reason, it is important to examine the deeper, unconscious processes contributing to the psychology of the balien.

I agree with Atkinson (1992) that it is necessary to be cautious in generalizing about all shamanism and that we should speak of *shamanisms* in recognition of its multiplicity of forms. Although I do not give priority to the role of performance and drama in my analysis of the Taman balien, I do take account of these aspects and think that they are essential to understanding the efficacy and sense of reality in balien ceremonies (see Chapter 7). Political power, however, seems to be far from the concerns of balien activities or the members of the balien group. (The possibility that balienism was once more closely related to power is discussed in Chapter 8.) And it would be difficult to convince me that anything about the Taman balien—ceremonial performance, ritual speech, illness, or therapy—is an expression of social protest, criticism, or commentary. I do not deny that these themes may be present in shamanism elsewhere in the world, but it would be misleading to apply them to the Taman.

Components for an Explanation of the Balien

Which approaches and perspectives are important in understanding Taman shamanism? First and foremost, I place Taman shamanism within the category of "medicine." This does not mean that Taman balien practices can be superimposed unreflectively over a Westernized model of medical practices or that they have the same meaning as medical treatments in Western society. Although the primary purpose of balien practices is defined as "curing" states of being thought of as illness, their meaning must be understood in the context of Taman society and culture. A balien's clients seek a healing service, not hunting magic, fortune-telling, or sacrificial propitiation.[1] Thus, from the point of view of the Taman villager, the balien is in a category that includes folk healers, trained medical practitioners, and others who dispense folk, patent, or pharmaceutical medicine. A sick person or the members of that person's family select either a balien or another kind of healer or medical practitioner. An example of a man's medical biography illustrates how for the Taman the balien phenomenon is integrated into a medical field.

> A man named Ontah said that on three occasions he had been so sick that he believed he would die. In each case he was treated first in the public hospital, staying there and receiving medication until he gave up hope. The first time, when he was a bachelor, he even went to Pontianak for treatment in a hospital, being treated with medicine for worms, but to no effect. Next, he was treated by a Malay shaman, who gave him an amulet and captured his soul in the water. During the second spell of illness, in 1976, he had to spend three weeks in the hospital at great expense to him, even though his condition did not improve. The doctor held out no hope for him, so he returned home. Next, he was treated by a Malay *dukun* in Kedamin with a treatment called *tepas* (see Chapter 3). This treatment did not cure him either, so he went to a balien in his own village, who performed *bubut* and *malai,* and also treated him with *sangka'* (antidotes) in case he had been poisoned. In his most recent bout of illness he received injections about eight or nine times. He was also treated by a dukun before going to a balien. The *mengadengi* ceremony was performed for him. Although he told me that he had no intention of becoming a balien, he said that if his illness ever returned he would have no choice but to do so. By the time my fieldwork ended people in the village were saying that Ontah would soon be inducted as a balien.

Because balienism must be understood in the context of a broader ethnomedical domain, I devote Chapter 3 to a variety of medical practices and treatments that supplement or contrast with (if not oppose) the balien's methods.

The balien system, like the other folk-healing practices known to the Taman, is medical in the sense that it comprises socially organized and culturally understandable response to illness, suffering, and bodily harm. The system of knowledge underlying the balien institution fits the following statement from a philosophical treatise on the nature of medicine: "The skills and commitment of medicine are aimed at the restoration of human beings" (Pellegrino and Thomasma 1981: 64).

But there are many problems with viewing the balien system as medicine. Immediately following the statement just quoted, the authors write: "The concepts of health and disease are both biological and evaluational" (Pellegrino and Thomasma 1981: 64). Does this apply to the balien? Leaving aside the evaluational component of medicine, we may assume that the balien does not use the same models as trained doctors, but does the balien use any biological concept of disease? Baliens, like the lay members of Taman society, view biological malfunctioning as illness, and they may attempt to treat it. But their explanations, interpretations, diagnostic procedures, and treatments are based on the concepts of souls and spirits and the relations between them (see Chapter 4).

One must use care when comparing balien or other folk medical practices to external (Western) or academic (sociological or anthropological) models of medical systems because doing so invites misleading assumptions. To an important but limited extent, balien healing ceremonies are "medical events" (Pellegrino and Thomasma 1981) that focus on clinical encounters between the healer and the patient and in which the meaning of the illness is interpreted (Kleinman 1978). But likening the balien to a clinician is not entirely apposite, given that many cues to the interpretation of illness are obtained in soul-flight and a dialogue with spirits. Nor is there a complete disjuncture between the role of the individual patient and those of his or her family members in many balien ceremonies; at times, whole families are treated together, or several people in addition to the main patient may be treated in rapid succession. In sum, the concepts of medicine are necessary and potentially very useful in explaining Taman shamanism, but there is also a danger in using these concepts and in forcing data into categories that are alien or predetermined or that have premises and implications that are misleading when applied to the Taman.

To understand the status and identity of the balien, it is necessary to explain several symbolic transformations associated with the acquisition of this identity. In my analysis of the balien's identity I use both social-organizational and psychological approaches. The uneasy relationship between these two approaches to magic and ritual has been a continuing thread throughout the history of anthropology. While identity is influenced by social attributes and criteria, the internalization of the balien's identity cannot be reduced solely to the assumption of a socially expressed role. The problems that lead a person to become a balien are culturally explained as "illness," as of course are the problems directed to the attention of the balien. Becoming a balien is a solution to troubles having their roots in adaptation to everyday life. To function as a balien, it is not sufficient to be able to perform in certain ways; one must also accept a certain view about oneself and others—identifying with what it means to be a balien and relating to others in new ways. It is important to look at structural conflicts in explaining shamanism, as Lewis has done, but this approach does not allow a full understanding of the balien phenomenon. A psychological perspective can provide insight into the subjective, interior side of identity in both the balien and the potential balien.

Most anthropologists oppose a consideration of the role of individual psychological factors in explaining shamanism. Atkinson (1992: 311) exemplifies the majority view: She suspects that studies emphasizing psychological processes do so at the expense of social dynamics. This, Atkinson says, is "offputting to sociocultural anthropologists," as it implies "a reductionism of symbolism and ritual to psychobiological functions," which would be as erroneous as viewing marriage "solely as a function of reproductive biology." Atkinson appears to be suspicious of those who infiltrate sociocultural anthropology's disciplinary turf by sneaking in individual processes, as if they were unrelated to group processes and had no effect on them.

While the use of any kind of psychological explanation is contentious to sociocultural determinists, depth psychologies such as psychoanalysis are particularly anathema to most anthropologists.[2] It is difficult to understand why anthropologists seeking to explain human thought and behavior would deliberately exclude from consideration sources of information about psychological processes, pretending either that they are epiphenomena or that they are irrelevant to social institutions. Unconscious processes are often messy, and this messiness vitiates the clean elegance idealized by those favoring an empiricist, "hard science" approach to anthropology. But many anti-empiricist anthropologists share this uneasiness about individual psychology and prefer to view human experiences as cultural constructions. The casual rejection by mainstream anthropologists of individual psychology and the possible insights afforded by psychoanalytic theory suggest an unwillingness to consider potentially valid alternative explanations of their research findings.

The psychoanalytic concept of hysteria helps explain the phenomenon of balien recruitment, accounting for the behavior and practices surrounding the illnesses that lead a person to become a balien. These illnesses may be called *pais layu-layu* (pining-away illness) or *dawawa jalu* (captured by a being). Symptoms typically include seeing and being drawn to an imaginary person, feelings of love toward that person, sexual dreams involving the imaginary person as an aggressor, physical weakness and unexplained emotional displays, melancholia, dreams involving food, loss of appetite, and inability to eat because of disgust resulting from delusions or mental associations about food. Such symptoms suggest that the person's illness is the result of the attention of an aggressive and seductive spirit.

These symptoms and illnesses are central to the balien institution. But they cannot be explained by recourse to the literature of the Turner school on dramaturgical cultural symbolism (Turner 1967, 1968, 1969, 1974)[3]; nor does Lewis's (1971) approach to trance-cults as manipulations about social power in a struggle between the classes or sexes explain them. It is here that a psychoanalytic approach to the symbolic process in the expression of symptoms, epitomized by Otto Fenichel's classic treatise on *The Psychoanalytic Theory of Neurosis* (1945), becomes useful (see Chapter 5). Within this model, projection, dissociation, and somatization are particular mechanisms for defending the ego in repressing thoughts or desires that create anxiety.

A final aspect of my approach to Taman shamanism is that I stress its objects and material culture. The balien is identified by certain objects, most important of which are the stones, the instruments of the craft without which the balien cannot function. Some of the objects of the balien's profession adumbrate core symbols of the balien's identity, which may be analyzed in reference to Turner's (1967) outstanding contribution on the paradoxical nature of ritual symbolism. Other objects are exchanged between the clients and the balien; they may be used in making offerings to spirits or may remain with the balien as payment for the work.

The New Age Movement and the Problem of Belief

The ancient techniques of shamanism have recently made a comeback in public and intellectual life through an eclectic social movement called the New Age. Shamanism is seen as a natural alternative to Western or modern medicine. The person who not only undergoes but uses shamanistic techniques takes control of his or her own health rather than surrendering to a bureaucratic, mechanistic, and ultimately dehumanizing medical system. Shamanism also has appeal as a psychology, especially for the Human Potential Movement (a subset of the New Age), in that it eschews Cartesian mind/body dualism, uses altered states of consciousness, and cultivates internal powers that are believed to enhance personal growth. Within the feminist wing of the New Age movement, shamanism is appealing because of the prominence of goddesses, suggesting the potential for a nonpatriarchal religion.

New adaptations of shamanism, called neoshamanism or urban shamanism, have arisen. According to Kenneth Meadows (1991: 8–9), a spokesman for the new shamanism, modern men and women can practice certain exercises to become self-taught shamans. Through learning shamanism, according to Meadows, people can develop insight into others' characters, be released from the illusions of false beliefs that are limiting and enslaving, discover personal gateways to greater power and mastery over their lives, learn to cope with difficulties and avoid obstacles, discover their hidden potential, and improve their personal relationships.

While the New Age preoccupation with shamanism has often been based on a legitimate quest for enlightenment and self-improvement, there have also been some misuses; perhaps this explains why many anthropologists (including medical anthropologists) are put off by the study of shamanism. This is unfortunate: By ignoring the popularization of shamanism, anthropologists miss an opportunity to provide valid information about it, thereby leaving the field in the hands of those who prey on people's ignorance and gullibility. Shamanism remains a proper subject for anthropological investigation, and as a field of inquiry it has an unrealized potential to contribute to intellectual culture (Flaherty 1992: 213–215). The larger problem is that shamanism is inherently ripe with exoticism, esotericism, and mystification. Many kinds of shamanism, including Taman shamanism, are inherently deceitful, and it is doubtful whether this deceitfulness can be filtered out (see Chapter 7).

There are two main sources of mystification in Taman shamanism: The first is the materialization of stones and pebbles in healing ceremonies, the second is the assertion that a balien is pierced with metal hooks inserted into the fingertips and eyeballs during initiation.[4] These elements present a problem for the anthropologist seeking to explain or even describe shamanistic practices. Should the anthropologist say that shamanism is a fraud, or that it is real for the Taman because they believe it, or that perhaps it is real after all? Is the only choice between the hard materialism that rejects the possibility that shamanism has any validity and the slippery slope of "alternate realities"? The anthropologist studying shamanism should find a middle course between acceptance and skepticism by adopting the "believers' interest without adopting their blind faith," as well as adopting the "debunkers' questioning attitude without adopting their cynicism" (Neher 1990: 6).

The question of the reality of magic and ritual and the problems surrounding the uses of illusion, deception, and mystification are central in anthropological analysis. It is important to have an appropriate theoretical and methodological framework for understanding these phenomena. Byron Good has recently reviewed the problematic nature of the question of "belief" versus "knowledge" in medicine and has pointed out the inadequacies of empirical as opposed to interpretive approaches (Good 1994). Following the reasoning of those interpretive social scientists who question the possibility of objective knowledge (see Rabinow and Sullivan 1979), Good is broadly critical of "the empiricist theory of medical knowledge" emerging from rationalist and intellectualist traditions. I agree that empiricist strategies alone cannot explain all aspects of medicine as a sociocultural phenomenon and that contemporary biomedicine cannot be taken as an absolute baseline for medical reality and knowledge. An interpretive approach is required to explicate people's embodied experiences in healing rituals and the conceptual apparatuses underlying them; and the data of interpretive anthropology need not be held to the standards of verification and falsification relevant for empirical data. But interpretive approaches do not tell us everything we need to know about the sociocultural reality of ritual healing. Whatever the shortcomings of empiricist anthropology, it would be foolhardy to throw out the baby with the bathwater by giving up entirely on an empiricist outlook.

Consider the analogy between the transformation of stones in the balien's ceremonies and the transubstantiation of the Host in the Roman Catholic Mass. The participants in the Mass believe that the wafer placed in the supplicant's mouth actually is the body of Jesus Christ, and the question of whether the wafer "really" becomes the body of Christ does not bear empirical investigation. However, other questions concerning the wafer and its uses do bear empirical investigation and may contribute to an understanding of the ritual. For example, in a description of the Mass it is appropriate to include information about wafers, what they are made of, and whether or not they are actually placed in the mouths of supplicants by priests. Similarly, the full meaning of stones and hooks in balien ceremonies cannot be conveyed purely in materialist or behaviorist terms, but a complete analysis of the ceremonies requires data and questions about actual stones and hooks, not just the cultural dogma surrounding them.

Interpretivist methodologies are no guarantee against distortion. In abandoning empiricism the ethnographer does not differentiate between the basic sources of information that go into the making of an ethnography: observation, informants' statements, and one's own ideas. As a result it is often impossible to tell how reliably the ethnography describes the knowledge and practices of the society under study, and to what extent it has been colored by the ethnographer's own opinions, beliefs, and wishes.

The problems of deception and mystification are particularly entrenched in balienism. All baliens start their careers as patients; they have all undergone the ceremonies they now perform; and they have been cured of illness by other baliens who are now their associates. Their role changes from patient to practitioner in the course of the most elaborate balien ceremony. Under the circumstances, it is simplistic to characterize the balien as knowingly deceiving his or her patients.

Taman shamanistic practices make little sense outside Taman culture. (It would therefore be of dubious value to instruct non-Taman readers in how they could become baliens or otherwise use their methods.) Some rituals have a universally understandable intuitive meaning, but the culturally embedded meaning of the practice depends on a belief system relating a specific concept of spirits to a specific concept of souls.[5]

It is easy to dismiss some Taman healing procedures as humbug, and many Taman would agree. (Even baliens themselves, at the time of their initiation, express skepticism about the veracity of the balien's cures.) But the Taman would *not* agree that the balien is a humbug. Despite the introduction of modern medicine in Taman society, the balien's stone massage has endured and is usually the first course of action in the case of illness. More important, the institution of the balien has remained robust despite being part of a pluralistic field of medical care systems to which the Taman have access and among which they must choose. The traditional healers have not disappeared but have adjusted their roles to meet changing social realities. While the balien tradition remains strong, many other traditional institutions of Taman society have decayed, such as the system of hereditary rank, the position of the chieftain (*temenggung*), and traditional burial and funerary practices. The balien system continues to meet some important needs. It is more than an ideology; it is a part of living, cultural reality.

Given the contemporary interest in feminism, multiculturalism, and the New Age, I expect that the Taman balien tradition, or at least some aspects of it, may appeal to many readers. As a kind of traditional healing, it is about as far as it can be from Western medicine. Its use of stones, its domination by women practitioners, and its primal figure being an ancestral goddess only add to its appeal. It is not my intention in this book to assist readers in cultivating their own spirituality. However, I hope that anyone seeking factual information about such practices will find a reliable account here, and that this book will contribute to a critical understanding not only of Taman folk healing practices but of shamanism in general.

Notes

1. The balien's *menindoani* ceremony may also be conducted to separate the souls of the dead from the world of the living. However, I have never witnessed such an event. This function corresponds to the shaman's role of "psychopomp," mentioned by Hultkrantz (1978).

2. Psychoanalytic anthropology is not without prestige in American anthropology, though it does seem to be highly marginal. Within British anthropology, psychoanalytic approaches are scorned.

3. The major school of symbolic analysis in social anthropology follows an approach originated by the late Victor Turner, whose work was "directed to the examination of meaning in the context of action and experience," and who viewed "meaning as emergent through the concrete articulation of symbols in practice" (Kapferer 1991: 7; cf. Bell 1992).

4. Of course, piercing is not a physical or medical impossibility, but there is no empirical evidence that it is fully carried out. The only evidence that it actually occurs is in the verbal statements of participants and other informants.

5. Because my study is focused on Taman ethnology, it is not my intention to relate the stones or any other element of the balien's practice to analogous elements used by shamans elsewhere in the world. Magical stones figure in the shamanisms of several traditional peoples, including the Samoyed, Eskimo, Nootka, and Araucana (Eliade 1964), and Elkin (1977) has provided a valuable description of aboriginal Australian shamanism, in which stone use is central. Stones have a number of different meanings and usages in shamanism, most of which are similar to the balien's use of stones; however, I am not aware of any other form of shamanism in which stones are thought to come into being in the manner described here.

2

The Taman People, Their Customs, and Their Social Structure

Location and Relationship to Other Ethnic Groups

The Upper Kapuas (Kapuas Hulu) is a frontier regency in the heart of Borneo, in the furthest reaches of West Kalimantan. Within it lies the source of the Kapuas, the longest river in Indonesia. One of six regencies in West Kalimantan (area: 56,650 square miles, 146,760 square kilometers; 1986 population: 2,819,496), the Upper Kapuas is the least-developed and most traditional part of this province. With an area of about 11,500 square miles (30,000 square kilometers), its population in 1982 was only 138,280.

Putussibau, its capital, is located on the Kapuas River at the mouth of the Sibau River and is the last market town on the Kapuas River, 550 miles (900 kilometers) upriver from the modern capital city of Pontianak. Putussibau is predominantly Malay, but people from all over the archipelago—Javanese, Bataks, Ambonese, Menadonese—not to mention ethnic Chinese, also live there, having been sent by the government or a private firm, or arriving on their own to seek their fortunes.

For a mere subdistrict (*kecamatan*), Putussibau is immense, covering 3,230 square miles (8,375 square kilometers). But its population is minimal: only 21,526 persons, according to 1986 government statistics. Of that total, 5,495 reside in the capital town of Putussibau, with another 5,150 inhabiting five adjacent Malay hamlets, all easily accessible from the main road. Beyond this core in which half the people in the subdistrict live are several more rural villages—Malay villages at the riverside and Kantuk villages inland. Further upstream, along the banks of the Sibau, Kapuas, and Mendalam Rivers, one meets a distinct culture: the Taman. Unlike the other groups who live in this subdistrict but have their roots elsewhere, the Taman have their only true homeland here. However, many Taman live and work in Sarawak, and some educated Taman have been assigned to posts in other parts of Kalimantan.

13

Map 1 Southeast Asia

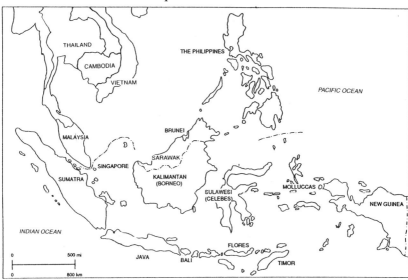

    The Taman villages can be divided into two branches or regencies, tra-
ditionally the domains of native suzerains called temenggung (an old
Javanese title): the Kapuas branch, which includes the Mendalam Taman,
and the Sibau branch.[1] Certain differences in vocabulary and other aspects
of dialect exist between the Kapuas and Sibau Taman, and there is even
slight variation within the Kapuas branch, but the dialects are mutually com-
prehensible.
    The Kapuas branch includes the villages of Suai, Melapi, Eko Tambai,
Siut, Lunsa Hilir, and Lunsa Hulu, which are between 2.5 to 14 miles (4 to
22 kilometers) from Putussibau. The Mendalam branch consists of but one
village, Semangkok, about 5 miles (8 kilometers) from Putussibau. The
Mendalam River is a tributary branching off from the Kapuas River between
Suai and Melapi. Semangkok is located upstream of Malay compounds and
downstream of several Kayan villages. The Sibau Taman live in two villages
(Sibau Hilir and Sibau Hulu), 4 to 9 miles (7 to 14 kilometers) from
Putussibau.[2] A few kilometers upstream of Sibau Hulu is Tanjung Lasa, an
unofficial village that does not have a headman. Most Taman villages are
divided into smaller units called *banua* (originally longhouses), which are
led by headmen; each has an average of about thirty households and under
200 members.
    According to 1987 government statistics, the total number of inhabi-
tants of all the Taman villages was 5,090. Of this number, approximately
4,500 were Taman—some 2,500 on the Kapuas, 1,700 on the Sibau, and 300
on the Mendalam. Making up the balance of the population were the Malay

Map 2 Political and Administrative Boundaries of Borneo

Map showing political and administrative boundaries of Borneo, with labels including KUDAT RES., WEST COAST RES., SANDAKAN RESIDENCY, SABAH, INTERIOR RES., TAWAU RES., BRUNEI, FIFTH DIV., FOURTH DIVISION, THIRD DIV., SIXTH DIV., SECOND DIV., FIRST DIV., SEVENTH DIV., BULUNGAN, BERAU, KALIMANTAN TIMUR, KUTAI, KALIMANTAN BARAT, KALIMANTAN TENGAH, KALIMANTAN SELATAN. Scale bar: 0, 100, 200, 300 km.

Legend:
— ·· — ·· International boundary
— · — · State boundary
·· —/ ···· Administrative boundary

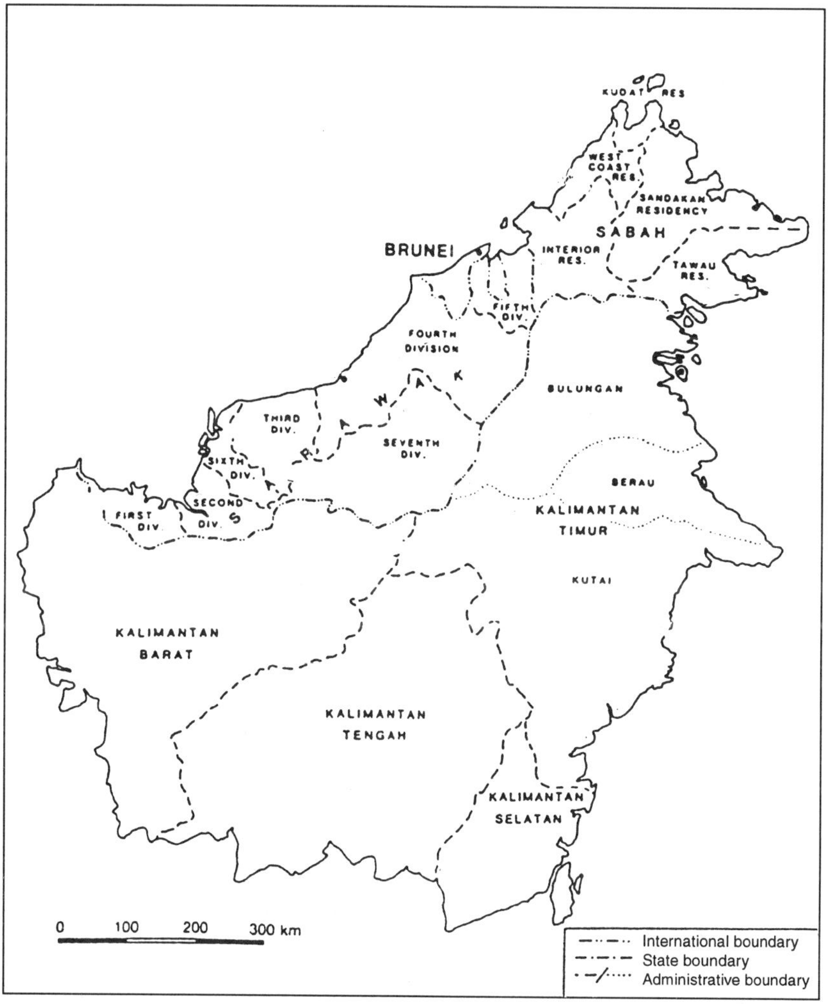

Source: Based on Rousseau 1990: xiv.

and, in significant numbers, the Kantuk and the Iban. Several Kantuk families moved to Siut around 1960, and in the late 1980s thirteen Kantuk households lived in their own compound slightly upstream of the village. An entire compound in Sibau Hulu is Iban; further upstream at Tanjung Lasa live a number of Kantuk as well as Bukat. Other nearby neighbors of the Taman are the Kayan, numbering under 1,000, who live in eight small villages upstream of Semangkok on the Mendalam River.[3] Beyond those villages is a Bukat settlement, Nanga Obat. Upstream of the outermost Taman village on the Kapuas are some recently formed villages of mixed ethnicity

Map 3 Upper Kapuas Regency, West Kalimantan, Indonesia

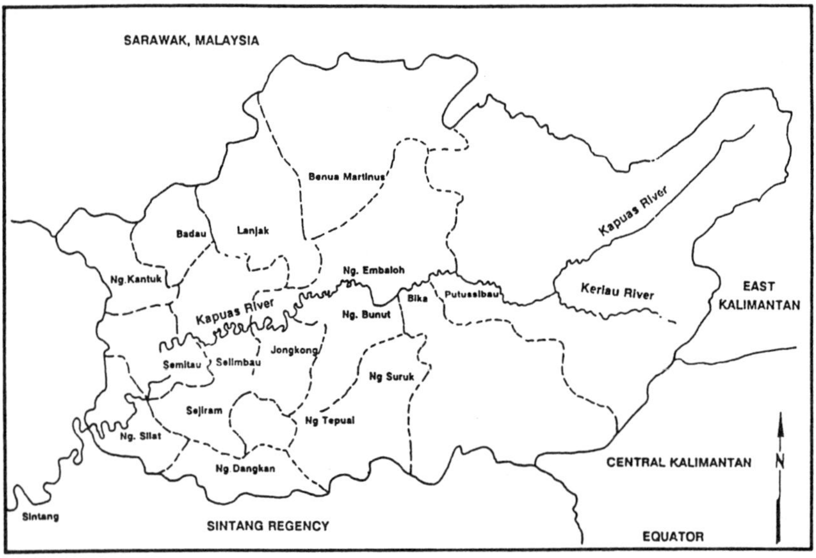

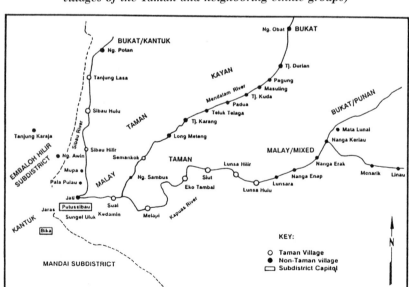

Source: Winzeler 1993: 172.

Map 4 Putussibau Subdistrict (showing locations of villages of the Taman and neighboring ethnic groups)

(mostly Malay)—Lunsara, Nanga Enap, and Nanga Erak—as well as a timber company.

Taman culture is close to but distinct from Putussibau town culture. Of the ten Taman villages, six can be reached on foot from Putussibau, except during those seasons when the ground is flooded. There are always some Taman villagers in town for such purposes as shopping, receiving medical treatment, selling produce, or attending school.

For the Dayak ethnic groups, the Malays represent the dominant and more cosmopolitan cultural majority.[4] Many Malay live in a manner similar to indigenous peoples such as the Taman and very often have Taman ancestors; some Malay also live in Taman villages. The Putussibau area is strongly Taman in ethnic origin, but people who have become Malay (*masuk Melayu*) by converting to Islam tend to forget or even deny this background. For example, a Sibau Taman who in his younger days had become a Muslim and moved to Putussibau opened a shop and eventually accumulated substantial wealth. In his sixties, this man became a hajji by making a pilgrimage to Mecca. He could be seen in Putussibau wearing the traditional Malay garb associated with a devout man. Rarely if ever did he visit his village, but when his landsmen visited his shop, he conversed with them in Taman.

Most conversions to Islam take place when a non-Muslim intends to marry a Muslim. An interesting but probably typical case occurred when a Malay man from Sarawak visited his family in a Taman village with his young son. Within days the son had become engaged to a girl from a family with a strong affiliation to the Kalimantan Evangelical Church. The family was so closely related by kinship ties to the Malay visitors that questions were raised about the appropriateness of the marriage; nevertheless, the girl's father agreed to the marriage, stating that as long as the customary bride-price was paid, she could marry the boy. The girl formally converted to Islam before the marriage ceremony, and she soon left the village, accompanying her new husband and father-in-law to Sarawak.

An overwhelming majority of the Taman speak the Upper Kapuas Malay dialect as well as Taman; standard Indonesian (Bahasa Indonesia) is understood by those who have gone to school or participated in a literacy program. In effect, almost all males speak or at least understand Bahasa Indonesia, but many females speak only Taman and Upper Kapuas Malay, because fewer females than males make sufficient progress in school to learn the national language. This has been the case since the introduction of education among the Taman. Few Taman, male or female, born before independence in 1949, completed primary school. But a large proportion of those born since 1960 have completed at least some elementary school, and there has been an ever-growing number of Taman youngsters attaining higher educational levels, including university.

Despite Indonesia's attitude of circumspection and rivalry toward

Malaysia (originating in a disastrous confrontation over Sarawak in 1963 and continuing with Indonesia's accusations of Communists infiltrating the Kalimantan border), the people of this area travel freely (if illegally) across the frontier. For them, kinship ties and opportunities for high-paying jobs and good, free health care override loyalties to arbitrary borders. The people of the Upper Kapuas feel a far stronger affiliation with Malaysia across the border than with other parts of Kalimantan, or in some cases, even with Pontianak. Taman often decorate their homes with objects obtained abroad, such as heavy brass lanterns from Brunei and garish, Warholesque portraits of themselves wearing jackets and ties or dresses.

In conclusion, contemporary Taman culture may be said to lie in the interface between older local traditions and the culture and norms of the outside world, including the nation-state.

Cultural and Linguistic Affiliations

The Taman are part of a larger ethnolinguistic entity identified by others (but not by themselves) as "Maloh" (Harrisson 1965; King 1985). Maloh refers to ethnic groups in the Embaloh Hilir, Embaloh Hulu, Mandai, and Putussibau subdistricts known as Embaloh (Tamambaloh), Kalis, Leboyan (Labiyan), Lauh (Alau), Palin (Apalin), and Taman. With the exception of the Taman, these names refer to the rivers where village compounds are located. Victor King (1985: 34–35) recognizes three major subgroups of the Maloh: Embaloh, Kalis, and Taman. He classifies the Leboyan, Lauh, and Palin as Embaloh, although he recognizes that there are substantial differences among them. The Taman, Embaloh, and Kalis dialects are not mutually intelligible, though they do share a great number of vocabulary terms. In details of custom they differ, too. Finally, these peoples commonly do not intermarry, although such intermarriage is totally acceptable. Apart from these differences, however, the Taman share with the Embaloh and Kalis a basic culture and form of social structure more so than they do with the Iban, Kantuk, Malay, and Kayan, who live in closer proximity. While their similar cultures and social structures are good reasons for maintaining the term Maloh, the Taman think of the Embaloh people, and not themselves, as Maloh, and say that the Maloh are Taman; conversely, the Embaloh call the Taman Embaloh (and probably Maloh). The Taman, Embaloh, and Kalis think of their own groups as primary and the others as derivative (Diposiswoyo 1985; King 1985).

More recently, S. Jacobus E. Frans L. (1992) identified as "Banuaka'" the peoples called Maloh by King. Like King, Jacobus wants to use a single term for these peoples in recognition of the similarities of their languages, customs, cultures, and societies. Jacobus prefers the term Banuaka' because it is used among the peoples themselves (especially the Taman) to refer to their own kind and to their land, society, people, and language. I agree that the term Banuaka' is preferable to Maloh, which the Taman people never use to refer to themselves. However, Jacobus's own examples show that the word Banuaka' is also not used across the board. Furthermore, while *banuaka'* is used in the Taman language to refer to the villages, people, and language of the Taman, and is perhaps used by Taman speakers to include people of the Tamambaloh, Leboyan, and other areas, it is not used to refer to ethnic identity. I find Jacobus's proposal of the term Banuaka' as an ethnonym intriguing, and in the absence of my own data either confirming or refuting it, I reserve judgment on his suggestion that the Taman people henceforth be called "Taman Banuaka'."

The Taman language has been classified by A. B. Hudson (1978) as "exo-Bornean," meaning that it appears to have closer affinities to languages indigenous to regions outside Borneo than to other Bornean languages. In a preliminary analysis Hudson (1970) had classed it as "Malayic Dayak" because of strong influences from the Malayic group of West Borneo, which appears to have originated in Malaysia and parts of Sumatra. However, Taman, Kalis, "Pari," and Embaloh (i.e., the languages of the Maloh, or Banuaka', peoples) have certain peculiarities that Hudson says are "definitely not Malayic and are, indeed, unique on the Bornean scene."[5] Hudson calls these languages "the Tamanic group" and makes a case for provisionally tracing them to Bugis. Recent research by Alexander Adelaar (1994) supports such a hypothesis.

Hereditary Rank

Stratification based on hereditary rank was previously an essential organizing principle in traditional Taman society. The conceptualization of people as *samagat* (noble), *pabiring* (middle rank), *banua* (commoner or freeman), or *pangkam* (slave) traditionally pervaded most aspects of Taman culture, leading King (1985) to make the rank system the centerpiece of his ethnographic and ethnohistorical study of the Maloh. Nor is such a pattern of social inequality in Borneo unique to the peoples comprising the Maloh/ Banuaka' complex. Jérôme Rousseau (1990) has discussed at length the principles and practices surrounding stratification throughout "Central Borneo." Although rank status no longer carries any weight in most social interactions, vestiges of this system persist in customs pertaining to marriage and divorce, and hence it does contribute to a person's status. For this reason a consideration of Taman social structure should begin with a description of some of the characteristics of the traditional rank categories.

Those occupying samagat status were symbolically associated with "goodness, health, and life" (King 1985: 93) by having their residences located at the upstream end of the village. Downstream of the village were the tomb huts (*kulambu*), in which (among the Embaloh) the coffins of the samagat and pabiring classes were placed on shelves above those of the banua. In former times, if people traveled to other villages, the samagat would sit in the middle of the boat and be propelled by oars manned by persons of lesser rank, and the use of umbrellas and parasols was prohibited by anyone but the samagat (Sungkalang 1982: 14).

The traditional perquisites of the samagat were such that they could impose fines on their villagers, and fines due to samagat were higher than those to others. Those who became indebted to the samagat might become debt slaves to them, subject to the whims of their masters (King 1985: 87). The free classes, too, were required to serve the samagat and offer them a portion of any game animals or of fish caught within village territory. The samagat occupied themselves with trading expeditions and visits to other villages and did not have to bother with agricultural labor.

Only the samagat could own slaves, who could be sacrificed both in house-building ceremonies and upon their master's death to accompany him as servants in the land of the dead. Slaves were obtained either as war captives or as the result of indebtedness. Those slaves captured in war could be exchanged for goods. Although slavery was abolished by the Dutch in the 1890s, King cites references to slaves as late as 1920. In present times a person can be fined for referring to someone as pangkam or suggesting that someone is pangkam.

The commoners (banua) were and are the majority of the citizenry of Taman villages. Traditionally their movement and the selection of land for cultivation by them were controlled by the samagat. The pabiring (middle rank) is seen by King as a residual category with no distinct role.

The prerogatives of high rank lasted longer than did slavery, but over the years there has been a breakdown in the meaning of the entire rank system, such that it is now virtually irrelevant socially. The decline of the rank system is part of the inexorable process of modernization that the Dutch tried to introduce through government and the church. The nationalist independence movement, which embraced a socialistic ideology, also hampered the traditional claims of class privilege. In modern Indonesian politics, with its egalitarian ideology of *Pancasila* (Watson 1987), the system of hereditary rank is abhorrent. This national ideology is an intrinsic part of the Indonesian education system. In contemporary society education is far more important than rank in determining a person's status, because a better-educated person is more likely to obtain a salaried job. By the late 1980s there was no positive correlation between education and rank among the Taman; there was perhaps even a negative correlation. Several samagat families possessed large old houses and great heirlooms, but others lived in dire poverty; meanwhile, a number of banua families also had large houses, and their children were better positioned to advance their lives.

King, who studied the Maloh in the 1970s, is correct in saying that the issues surrounding rank have not disappeared entirely. The attitude evinced by samagat that they are superior to other Taman and are rightful leaders is resented if not scorned by the non-samagat majority. Nevertheless, a reader could get an exaggerated sense of the importance of rank in contemporary Maloh society from King's account.

The main consequences of the rank system in contemporary society are in marriage payments and in fines involved in divorce and adultery. The payments and fines of parties of the samagat stratum are double those of the other strata of society. The middle rank (pabiring) has lost whatever distinct meaning it once had, since marriage payments for persons of that rank are the same as those for the banua rank. In contemporary society, in which leadership is by headmen who are appointed by consensus, a person's position within the traditional system of rank carries little weight. Marriages are not endogamous within ranks, so there is no castelike purity.

Village Structure

The traditional Taman village was a single longhouse (*langko soo*) containing as many as twenty-five apartments. Longhouse villages were not only an architectural style but an integral part of the traditional way of life for the majority of Dayak tribes. Following independence in 1949, the Indonesian government put pressure on villagers to move out of longhouses, and in much of Kalimantan traditional longhouse villages have been replaced by single-family dwellings. This anti-longhouse policy has since been reconsidered, however, and the Dayak longhouse is now recognized as a valuable facet of the nation's cultural heritage. Taman villages today consist of a combination of longhouses and individual houses; about half of the people live in each kind of residence.

The contemporary village has evolved from its earlier form. Traditional Taman villages were located near the riverbanks, as villages are to this day, but structures were built on extremely high posts because of the threat of raids by enemy tribes such as the Kantuk and Kayan. Modern longhouses are lower than traditional ones, they tend to have narrower verandas, and they incorporate modern materials.

The longhouse community comprises individual households that build their apartments according to their own tastes, needs, and abilities. Materials used in building the longhouse range from ironwood to corrugated zinc to bark. Rarely is a unified design sustained for the entire length of a structure. The longhouse veranda cannot be considered communal property because the rights of the people who live behind a particular portion of veranda space should be respected. However, in large ceremonies, not only is the veranda used communally, but partitions separating the outer rooms of the apartments are removed to make room for the guests.

In the traditional longhouse the noble (samagat) class families inhabited the upstream end of the longhouse, and the headman, who was also of noble rank, lived in the apartment at the head of the house. To some extent this traditional pattern is still followed, but nowadays the headman need not be of noble rank, he may have his own individual house, and in some cases not only does he not occupy the upstream end of the building, but his own apartment may have no visible signs of wealth and may be in disrepair.

Schools and houses for teachers have been built in every village complex, and some teachers are imported from remote parts of Indonesia. Education has introduced bureaucratic routinization into village life. Schools are in session from Monday to Saturday at specified hours. During periods of intensive agricultural work, there is forbearance about progress in schoolwork, and in some villages pupils are expected to assist in the agricultural labor at the teachers' own fields. Besides academics, scouting (*pramuka*) and volleyball are important school activities.

In some larger villages entrepreneurs have set up shops, often licensed by the local government. These are foci of village activity; it is here that people buy and sell rice, depending on the season. Men bring in rubber to be weighed and buy cigarettes with the proceeds. These shops operate on a credit system and obtain their supplies from distributors in town.

Another focus of activity in some villages is the church. Catholic chapels have been built in several Taman villages, and Sunday services are led usually by a teacher. Most of the congregants are women and children.

Kinship System

The Taman have a cognatic kinship system; the bilateral kindred is the focus or basis of each person's reference group (cf. Appell 1976). The family system is based on a "stem family" unit: that is, ideally, one child will bring his or her spouse into the domestic unit and raise their children there; the other siblings will marry out. The person who stays is sometimes thought to be "mother's favorite" and may stay out of loyalty to the parents. Bringing a spouse to live in the parent's residence is called *piring toa,* meaning that that child supports the parents. Sometimes, however, two siblings will raise their families within the parental home. This could cause unbearable stress if, as is the case among the Iban, the "*bilek*-family," to use Freeman's (1958, 1970) terminology, farmed one plot, then accusations about the in-law not carrying his or her share of the work could arise. Among the Taman, however, adult siblings living together in a bilek-family each farm their own plots. Husbands and wives may in fact be in charge of cultivating their own individual plots, although the different members of the family will work together. Couples with unmarried children living together within a bilek-family thus have their own property, but these joint households are in a significant sense "units of consumption" because they share one hearth.

The main heirlooms—gongs, cannons, antique porcelain jars (if any), and traditional clothing—stay within the bilek-family; however, when a child marries out, that child is given a reasonable share in consideration of the fact that he or she forfeits the right to inherit the house and rights in land, including agricultural lands and rubber groves. (With five or more children typically marrying outside the bilek-family, many offspring of poorer families do not inherit any significant heirlooms.) If the child later divorces and returns to the natal bilek-family, these heirlooms are returned.

Customary Law

The Taman are keenly interested in their customary law, which concerns disputes, marriage, and sexual relationships. As the Taman see it, their customary legal code (*adat*) is the essence of their social structure. Through a study of traditional legal tenets, we can understand the ideology of Taman social structure, especially the systems of rank and gender relations. Taman law is based on a system of fines intended to compensate for shame or hurt feelings. These fines uphold propriety about norms and respect, especially respect for the dead.

Marriage Payments

The system of marriage payments is the paradigm for the other domains of Taman adat law. Within Taman adat the male side and the female side are opposite and reciprocal categories.

For pabiring and banua, brideprice (*pekain*) may be paid in either money (Rp 110,000) or certain objects such as gongs, small cannons (bading) 1 *pikul* (62.5 kilograms or 138 pounds) in weight, beads, shawls, beaded clothes, gold, or antique silver coins. For samagat the bride-price is double this amount. (See Appendix D on the value of the rupiah.)

If the wife is taken away, a payment called *perabut* is added to the basic pekain. This payment is considered to be "in repayment of the mother's milk." It is comparable in value to pekain: Rp 100,000, or two beaded suits (*manik lawang*), or a gong 1 *jengkal* (6 to 8 inches) in diameter or a cannon weighing half a pikul. As an alternative to perabut, the woman's parents may request that the man live with them for two to three years, a service called *lalangi*.

Pananga' is the term for an additional marriage payment on top of pekain required to marry samagat. If a samagat man marries a pabiring or banua woman, the man pays the pekain for samagat, and the woman pays back one-half of that to the man. If a samagat man marries a samagat woman, he pays the pekain for samagat. If a non-samagat man marries a samagat woman, he pays pananga' so that his children can become samagat. He himself remains non-samagat, as does the non-samagat woman who marries a samagat man. Even the offspring of such a marriage are not fully considered samagat unless they themselves marry into samagat status and pay a moderate fine called *menyelongi* to "cleanse" themselves (Anyang 1985: 99). The value of samagat status in contemporary Taman society does not inhere in the individual person but rather in the person's ability to confer this quality to his or her descendants. Bride-price is also paid (or returned) in the case of divorce if one party is determined to be at fault.[6]

Nonmarital Sex

The Taman are not especially puritanical about sex, but they vigorously regulate sexual behavior with legal sanctions. Sungkalang, an eloquent spokesman for Taman values, has this to say about extramarital sex resulting in pregnancy:

> The occurrence of an unmarried or widowed woman getting pregnant not by her husband is forbidden and culpable. Usually the woman will admit only after examination or interrogation that she has committed an indecent act with a man, causing her to become pregnant. Such a pregnancy, besides becoming the focus of public discussion, may also result in an adverse situation for the members of society, in the form of nonstop rain disturbing the work of the people, especially swidden agriculture. Therefore it is in society's interest to resolve the situation [by prosecuting the couple] so that normal conditions may return. (Sungkalang 1982: 95; trans. JHB)

A man's sexual activity is always legally culpable except with his own wife. Female sexual behavior is regulated; the use of the female by the male must be compensated. (Homosexuality is unheard of and is apparently incomprehensible to the Taman.)

Traditional law has it that if an unmarried man enters an unmarried woman's sleeping space, only after three nights does the woman's father

> advise the youth to be responsible for whatever happens. If he does not heed this advice he is subjected to a fine called *kesopan orang tua,* amounting to two *kelitau. Kelitau* means slave. In about 1932 . . . this fine was standardized so that one *kelitau* equaled 15 Dutch rupiahs. . . . If he persists he is fined again, unless he promises to marry the girl. In this case, usually it is not adultery but only a phase of getting to know each other. (Ali As 1967: 19; trans. JHB)

Nowadays the traditional custom of the father waiting three nights is no longer upheld. The father or any other male relative will confront the young man and probably beat him. The offense is called *meraja* or *badak*. Intercourse even between engaged people is punishable.

Young, unmarried men claim that they do steal into their girlfriends' sleeping space enclosed with mosquito nets. This is of course a very tricky business, involving such feats as creeping over rafter beams in a longhouse or standing for hours under the house, in the cold night air, amid the mud and other refuse. Those instances in which a man boldly enters without invitation are likely to end in disaster, especially if the woman does not desire him. Additional penalties also apply if the illicit relationship is considered incestuous.

A distinction is made in Taman law between fornication (illicit but consensual intercourse) and rape; both are culpable but the former is less so. Worse than either, however, is adultery. In addition to other fines, the wronged parties must be compensated in the amount of half of their marriage payments. Certain fines are paid not only to the aggrieved spouses but to the unfaithful woman's parents and the council of adat elders who adjudicate the case. A still higher fine is demanded if a woman becomes pregnant outside of marriage. These fines vary depending on the particular village.

Death and Burial

Another focus of customary law pertains to death. The ceremonialism of funerals usually far exceeds that of weddings; furthermore, only in funerals are guests expected to bring gifts, which are publicly acknowledged. After the body has been buried, a period of prohibition (*buling*) is observed within the longhouse or village unit (banua) of the bereaved family. Buling lasts ten days among the Sibau Taman and fifteen days among the Kapuas and Mendalam Taman; it is a period of circumspect behavior during which time music should not be played and no one may wear watches, gold jewelry, or traditional fine garments. For violating buling a person is fined ten *bua'*, an amount equivalent to Rp 6,000. The full penalty is enforced only if the liable person has prior knowledge that buling is being observed; if buling has been violated inadvertently, the fine is reduced by half.

If a person is widowed, a conference of elders is held to determine whether that person should observe a one-year period of mourning during which he or she not only may not marry but must observe all the restrictions of buling and other prohibitions on drinking liquor, combing the hair or using hair tonic, eating mushrooms and certain kinds of meat and fish, and looking up at the sky.

Minor improprieties are also resolved in fines. For example, if the corpse of a person who did not live in a particular longhouse is brought inside, a small fine called *sut* or *sengkalan* is paid. A person building a house may not attend a funeral, and if a family member of someone attending a funeral is abroad, the person visiting the funeral is paid sengkalan.

Elaborate ceremonies for the departed spirits, called *mulambu membir kulambu,* are no longer practiced (see Sastrowardoyo et al. 1983/1984: 105; Harrisson 1965: 275–287), nor is secondary burial (*menolang*). According to Jacobus, corpses were reburied either because the original burial place was destroyed by a natural disaster or because of recurring dreams of the person's descendants (Jacobus 1992: 15).

Agama Jolo: Customary Religion and Origin Myth

"Religion" (*agama*) in Indonesia refers to monotheistic world religions, in contrast to traditional local beliefs (*kepercayaan*) and associated rituals. The Taman, however, speak of customary beliefs as *agama jolo* (the old religion). Agama jolo consists of stories about ancestral deities who created the world, subsequent spirits that must be propitiated, and beliefs concerning the human soul and the afterlife. Apart from shamanism, practices that would fall under the rubric of agama jolo include bird omenism, the propitiation of spirits in agriculture and house building, and mortuary practices. The Taman people have no priestly role or organized priesthood. While traditional cosmology is animistic, it incorporates a notion of a creator God, Alatala, and a judge of the dead, Yang Suka, who is also equated with God.[7]

According to the Taman creation myth, as described by Balunus (n.d.), Alatala created heaven, the earth, and the sea, as well the various ancestral gods and goddesses who have dominion over them. These three worlds are arranged vertically, with heaven on top, the sea on the bottom, and earth in between; each world consists of seven layers. Heaven is controlled by the sun (Mata'aso), the moon (Bulan), the stars Iyangpani' (the Aldebaran?), Bintangtalu (Orion), Balunus (the Pleiades), Grandmother Ambong (the goddess of rice), and various other spirits. Among these are the couple Grandfather Kunyanyi' and Grandmother Sampulo, who created mankind (*mintuari*) out of yellow clay taken from the deepest layer of the earth. Underneath heaven is the earth, and under the earth is the sea, a lower world ruled by such gods and goddesses as Kindanum (Tindanum), Juata, and Gana, as well as other spirits.

After some false starts, the first human being created by Grandmother Sampulo was a man, Idiilangilangsuan; next, a woman, Ina', was created. Early people were forced to retreat to a mountaintop following a great flood (*ai bah*) that covered the whole world. The people had no food so mushrooms (*kulat basi*) found growing on the mountain were collected and eaten. The mushrooms were intoxicating, and after eating them, people could no longer speak or understand the same language. As a result, the various races and nationalities of the world differentiated from one another, all speaking different languages.[8] Some years later the floods returned, killing many people. Among those who survived were Grandfather Sapinangsalowe, along with his wife, seven sons, and one daughter. Grandfather Sapinangsalowe planted crops to provide for his family and then built a boat in which he traveled the world with his sons. He was the first person to travel the world "up to the edge of the sky," and he became rich from his travels. Following his voyage, he returned to his village to lead his people, the Taman, and he gave them their adat.

The Status of Introduced Religions

Since Indonesia's independence, those people unaffiliated with a major religion have been encouraged to join one for purposes of identification. For example, it is necessary to state a child's religion for that child to enter school. Both Islam and Christianity tend to denigrate as "devil worship" the traditional animistic beliefs and practices (including shamanism) common throughout Borneo. For the most part the Taman have joined Christian churches that are relatively tolerant of customary ways of life that include sacrifices to spirits and festive drinking.

Roman Catholicism was introduced to the Taman by the Dutch fathers in the 1930s. The Catholic Church was very active in developing education, and its work accounts for almost all of the education of Dayak people in the Upper Kapuas beyond the elementary level. It operates junior and senior secondary schools as well as a girls' dormitory. Until the 1970s only a minority of Taman people had become Catholic. Presently, most of the Taman on the Kapuas are Catholic. In Siut, Melapi, Semangkok, and Lunsa, in particular, the great majority of residents are Catholic. These villages all have Catholic chapels; and the Dutch and U.S. pastors based in Putussibau make rounds occasionally to serve their flock.

Protestantism was introduced by the Kalimantan Evangelical Church (Gereja Kalimantan Evangelis), a church evolving out of Lutheran and Calvinist missions entering Borneo as early as 1835, but reaching the Upper Kapuas only in 1972. In 1974 a congregation was founded in Sibau Hilir, but as Moses Siong (1984) writes, support for the congregation has only been incidental. The Evangelical church is aware that many Dayak people in the Upper Kapuas are Roman Catholic; its main concern is to reach the remaining unaffiliated people before they turn to Islam. At times Sibau Hilir has had a minister and a motivator from this church. A boys' dormitory is run by this church for pupils from the villages studying in Putussibau. About half the villagers in Sibau Hilir and Sibau Hulu are Protestant, while Tanjung Lasa has a Protestant majority. In the same way that some Taman longhouses were converted en masse to Catholicism in the early 1970s, others came to the Protestant faith under the leadership of their headmen.

The New Tribes Mission, a U.S. Fundamentalist Baptist Church, has stationed two missionary families in Eko Tambai to proselytize to the Taman. Unlike the Catholics, they work in the Taman language. They lead classes in several villages on the Kapuas, and while they have converted a core of committed adherents, the sheer precedence of the Catholic Church in the area has relegated them to secondary status. Affiliated with these missionaries is the Mennonite Church (Gereja Muria), which receives foreign backing. The Gereja Muria established a church in Putussibau in the 1970s, led by an Ambonese minister.

A small fraction of the Taman population, mainly older people, have never converted to a world religion and are considered animist; however, they seem to be no more animistic than the Catholics and Protestants. An even smaller fraction of the Taman are Muslim. (An Islamic prayer house has been built in Sibau Hilir but is never used.) A considerable number of Taman people have converted to Islam, but no longer consider themselves Taman.

Economic Life

Like most rural Southeast Asians, the Taman consider themselves to be above all else cultivators and consumers of rice, and identify themselves as farmers (*petani*). Shifting cultivation is arduous work with little profit, but there is a visceral feeling among the Taman that families must cultivate rice, regardless of its seeming lack of economic rationality. As one informant said, what needs to be avoided is the humiliation of being descended upon by guests and not being able to feed them. But it is rare indeed that a family's rice harvest can feed even the family for a whole year, much less guests.

The choice of a spot for cultivation is based on the observation of stars and of the flight patterns of seven sacred species of birds known as *burung antis*. Trees are cut down and left to dry for over a month during the hot and (it is hoped) rainless season before the entire field is set on fire. Remaining burnable material is gathered into mounds for reburning. Meanwhile, cooperative work groups are organized in which a row of people (usually men) puncture the ash-covered land with sharpened sticks while a succeeding row (usually women) fill the holes with rice seeds. Several varieties of rice are planted; maize, squash, cucumbers, and mustard greens may be cultivated along with rice. Once the heavy rains have begun, the back-straining and headache-inducing work of weeding must soon begin, followed, as the crop matures, by a period when someone from the family must be on the grounds at all times to guard against animal as well as human predators. In anticipation of the harvest, special sheds and mats must be made to dry out the fresh-cut rice plants. Again, cooperative work groups are organized to cut and carry the crop. The rice is dried out and threshed, then put into baskets (each load weighing 100 pounds or more) and carried by members of the work group from the rowboat to the village. There it is further processed to remove the hull, winnowed, and stored.

In March, after the harvest and when the price is low, villagers might sell their rice to merchants in the village to buy necessary consumer items such as soap, noodles, biscuits, canned fish, cigarettes, tobacco, salt, sugar, coffee, fuel, and cooking oil. These village shops charge prices higher than those in town. In this way stocks of hundreds of kilograms are depleted within a few months, until the same villagers who sold rice are forced to buy it at prices as much as 100 percent higher than what they received for their hard-earned crop. It is estimated that by growing rice in this way, a farmer earns the equivalent of Rp 300,000 to Rp 600,000. A bad crop could be worth as little as Rp 100,000.

Even an excellent crop worth Rp 1,000,000 would not satisfy the economic needs of a large family because the crop must be not only consumed by the family but also traded for consumer goods. Rice is the main component of every meal in a Taman home. For example, a family of eight consumes one *gantang* (2.5 kilograms) and five *mok* ("mugfuls") of rice a day—nearly 3 kilograms.[9] Their basic needs cost Rp 65,500 a month: Rp 4,000 for spices such as onions and garlic; Rp 5,000 for cooking oil; Rp 3,000 for petroleum oil for household use; Rp 1,000 for salt; Rp 9,000 for sugar; Rp 5,000 for coffee; Rp 3,500 for soap; Rp 17,000 for school fees for two children attending junior high school in Putussibau; an average of Rp 15,000 on clothes (if each person buys three sets of clothes a year); and Rp 3,000 for tobacco. The family of eight that eats 3 kilograms of rice a day would need 1,095 kilograms (about 2,400 pounds) of rice a year just for them to eat. Once their rice is gone, they have to buy it at prices much higher than what they received for their own rice.

Rice cultivation is not the only economic occupation of the Taman. In the late 1980s, when the price of rubber was very high, it was possible for able-bodied people (especially children) to earn up to Rp 10,000 a day by tapping rubber. Selling fruit from door to door can also be a useful though not very lucrative occupation. In recent years women from some Taman villages have gone to town to market vegetables from their fields and gardens, wild fruit such as durians, rambutans, longans, and mangosteens, and wild mushrooms, in season.

Chickens and ducks are commonly raised for sale, pigs less so, and some people also raise cattle as emergency capital; they are slaughtered at funerals to feed guests and are sold in case a large amount of money is needed at once. For example, a man who was sued for having an illicit liaison with a married woman that resulted in the birth of a child sold a calf to raise some money when it was determined that he would have to pay adat fines because of the baby, even though it had died. He had already liquidated most of the rest of his assets in paying all the other adat fines that had followed his grievous action. Fortunately for him, he had extended credit to many people, so by collecting these debts he was able to get back on his feet. But another man was permanently ruined economically by the loss of his cattle, some of which were slaughtered by him and others of which were killed by bandits.

Young men especially hunger for the chance to go to Sarawak, where the wages of even menial labor allow them not only to provide for their families but to buy speedboat motors, tape recorders, and nice clothes. They also provide the capital necessary to buy gongs, that is, to marry. Logging is popular and potentially lucrative (but hazardous) work for men. People with carpentry or mechanical skills can do very well for themselves; one such man goes to Sarawak occasionally to work and does no farming at home. Women, too, can find opportunities for work in Sarawak.

Notes

1. The title and role of the temenggung as functionary leaders of the ethnic group were first given to Taman customary leaders under Dutch colonial rule in 1918 (Diposiswoyo 1985: 120).

2. *Sibau* is a Taman word for the rambutan fruit. *Hilir* and *hulu* are Indonesian terms, referring to downstream and upstream, respectively. Sibau Hilir means Lower Sibau and Sibau Hulu means Upper Sibau. The Taman names for these villages are, respectively, Banua Sio Ilutang and Banua Sio Ira'ang.

3. The West Kalimantan Kayan are only a portion of a much larger ethnic group whose homeland is in Sarawak and East Kalimantan (Rousseau 1990).

4. "Dayak" refers here to people who identify with any indigenous ethnic group in Kalimantan or Sarawak. The term also may refer to any and all non-Muslim native peoples of Borneo. Catholics outnumber Muslims by 50.1 percent to 44.8 percent in the Putussibau subdistrict, though not in the Upper Kapuas as a whole, where more than 54 percent are counted as Muslims.

5. The term "Pari" was coined by O. Von Kessel in 1850 to refer to several different Dayak groups (King 1985: 37), but in this context it probably refers only to the Embaloh (King 1985: 210).

6. Divorce is rather common among the Taman. Siong (1984) surveyed 186 families of all religions in Sibau Hilir. In these families, 30 (16.1%) of the heads of households had been divorced. A wide variety of reasons are given for divorce, and it is not always possible to identify one spouse as blameworthy; often conflicts between in-laws set the stage for the termination of marriage.

7. The word "Alatala" or a cognate is very often found among Dayak peoples. The accepted scholarly view is that this word is adapted from the Arabic expression *Allah-ta-ala* (God most high) but without the doctrinal implications. Another name for God is Sampulo Padari.

8. The flood legend, as recounted by Diposiswoyo, is used by the Taman to explain why they lost the art of writing. Unlike the other peoples of the world, the Taman wrote on their loincloths, and when the flood came, these were lost in the water. They were later retrieved, but when they were left out to dry in the sun, they were swept up in the air and became birds. The writings of the Arabs and Chinese were preserved, but only in a damaged form, having been disfigured by the water. Only the white man's writing was unharmed by the flood (Diposiswoyo 1985: 64–65).

9. This figure is well in line for people who subsist mainly on a rice diet. King (1985: 171) estimates the average consumption of rice per person at slightly over a pint per day; this of course varies according to age and sex.

3

Therapeutics, Pharmacopoeia, and Medical Pluralism

In Taman village society, treatment by a balien is usually the first response to symptoms of illness. In some cases, serious illnesses are treated only by baliens until they are resolved. But the balien does not function in a vacuum, and a sick person is often treated, over the course of an illness, by several different kinds of people, including doctors and nurses as well as folk healers. The balien treats illness on the presumption that it was crafted and sent by a spirit. The balien's healing power does not depend primarily on the use of any medicines but on special instruments and direct negotiation with spirits. This chapter describes the range of medicinal and other therapeutic treatments existing alongside balien practices, as well as the status of modern medicine in Taman society. It also addresses the uses of medical knowledge and attitudes toward it among the Taman.

The folk-medical practices described in the first sections of this chapter are part of everyday knowledge, or are not integrated into complex systems. Even the more secretive and esoteric traditional healing practices involving medicines and other objects are carried out by those who are considered not healers but simply people who possess and know how to administer particular substances.

Only one type of healer, the Malay dukun, has a professionalized role as a specialist, even though other people who use their knowledge or materials in their possession to cure illnesses may demand compensation.[1] Although there are various kinds of dukuns, their role and general approach to healing is well understood by the Taman. Using a combination of herbalism and Islamic knowledge, they represent a different folk-medical paradigm from that of the balien, and they are a frequently patronized alternative.

"Village Medicine"

A range of medical alternatives is available to the Taman, evidence of the cultural pluralism of the Upper Kapuas area. A general division is recognized between "village medicine" (*obat kampung*) and cosmopolitan medicine, called "government medicine" (*obat pemerintah*) by some. Diseases caused by either human or spirit agents are considered inherently incurable by government medicine. "Village illnesses" must be cured with village medicine. Ordinarily people do not speak openly about the medicines they have. There are two explanations for such secrecy: The first is that knowledge or ownership of an antidote implies ownership of poisons or knowledge of their manufacture. The second reason is that a person who has medicine may feel an onerous obligation to cure others. In cases of illness, people often do not offer the medicines they possess, to avoid getting involved. If a person's possession of medicine becomes known, that person will be expected to help.[2] In short, medicine and pharmacological knowledge are subjects about which many people are uncomfortable.

An exception to the above statement is a knowledge about common medicinal plants, which are cultivated in gardens or grow naturally in the village or swidden fields. They are made into medicaments used in treating illnesses caused by an organic condition. They have largely been replaced with pharmaceutical medicines.

Bunga randi' (Hibiscus rosa-sinensis) is commonly used to draw pus out of infections. *Tarangga (Impatiens* cf. *balsamina)* is crushed and applied as a salve on wounds. Many people are aware of the use of *serunggan* (*Cassia alata*) for fungal itch, though few people have confidence in its effectiveness. *Langka (Artocarpus heterophyllus,* the jackfruit) leaves can be burnt and rubbed into ulcerated sores as medication.

Several medicinal plants are thought to cure stomach problems as well, among them *urat inyak,* roots of the coconut palm (*Cocos nucifera*) boiled in water and drunk as a cure for dysentery. A remedy for sharp abdominal pain is to rub the ashes of the bark and perhaps leaves of the *lukai* (*Annonaceae*) tree on the stomach. The burning of these materials is supposed to frighten off the spirits that cause this illness.

Some other medicines, not as commonly known, include leaves or seeds of the *rambean* tree (*Baccaurea motleyana*) boiled, and the water used for eyedrops. *Limpa dutana (Lindernia viscosa)*, a weed found in swidden fields, is boiled and drunk for respiratory tract ailments and also malaria. The flower *bunga kayu* (unidentified) is used to treat chicken pox and measles.[3] *Reak (Imperata cylindrica)*, a very common weed found in disused fields, is boiled and drunk to prevent the return of illness.

Some simple therapies involve no use of medicine. To rid the body of wind that causes headaches, colds, and flu, one pours saltwater on the chest and pinches the skin until a red mark is visible. People may create patterns in this manner, and some youths use this technique to spell out the titles of pop songs or phrases like "I love you." To cure headaches the temples may also be pinched; another technique is to draw a cloth band around the head, twisting it as if tightening a vise.

Painting a circle, a cross, or another pattern on an ailing body part, using lime (sometimes mixed with turmeric or chewed betel leaves), turmeric, or red onions, is a simple therapy for a variety of pains such as sore throats, headaches, abscesses, or toothaches. This treatment, called *pusau,* is common in the Taman villages and was learned from the Malay dukuns. People who know the fine points of this practice recite the Arabic incantation "*Bismillahir rohmanir rohim*" ("In the name of Allah the compassionate, the merciful"). Others who do not thoroughly understand the blessing commonly mispronounce it. The pusau blessing has other uses besides curing illness. A ceramic jar for fermenting liquor may be painted with a cross to strengthen its contents, and women may use a pusau of lime and betel water to make themselves irresistible to men.

Uncommon Medicines

The medicines just described have no economic value as commodities: They are free to anyone who finds or grows them. Similarly, simple home therapies have no compensation value. But less common medicines are either kept secret or used for economic gain; payment is demanded either because the product itself is scarce or because expertise is required to activate its powers. More advanced knowledge of medicinal plants—the effect of combining plants and the acquisition of difficult-to-find plants from the forest—is declining among the Taman. The children of people knowledgeable about such medicines have no interest in learning about them, and people who own these medicines do not let others use them or know about them.

Animal products such as porcupine quills and the fat and gallbladders of bears are kept for medicinal uses such as the treatment of chest pains (*najam*).

A stone, *Batu Arang* ("coal stone," possibly petrified charcoal or bark), is medically useful in treating wounds. It is found rarely in the forest, and is considered very valuable. People may buy and sell it (a price of Rp 10,000 was mentioned), or keep it hidden. One day a girl was bitten on the toe by a centipede. News spread quickly through the village and a neighbor provided Batu Arang to treat it. The toe was tied in a tourniquet, and the stone was put on top of the wound. One man brings his Batu Arang to a lumber concession and treats men injured by falling wood, charging them a quantity of rice or anything else he can trade.

A significant source of uncommon medicines is dreams.

Pulok showed me a kind of vine he keeps wrapped up that he got from the top of a tree. Before he found it he had a dream: An old man with a long beard said "I'm giving this thing to you, grandson. Go to the place and I'll show it to you." After this dream he found the vine. Then he had another dream in which he met the same old man, who told him that the vine had many uses: (1) To be able to have many children, and (2) So as not to have any more children. The vine can be cooked in water and drunk to cure several illnesses.

He has never given any to anyone because no one knows he has it, but he added that if someone asked him for some he might give it to them. He is very proud of this vine, and says, "It's not that I saw it, I dreamed of it."

Pulok's reluctance to use his medicine to help others is typical of the Taman attitude. A male informant with whom I had worked closely for several months, and who was helping me to assemble a herbarium, said that knowledge of medicine was secret, because if you have it you must share it. He said that people who have or know about medicine do not mention it unless they can profit from it. On another occasion, a man said that "people do have medicines but do not want to admit it. They keep them for their own needs. If you ask they won't give it." Pulok himself, who had a remarkable assortment of medicines (see below) said when I prompted him that he had a cure for leprosy (a prayer from a book, recited over some wood), but he did not want to use it to help a man in the village who suffers from that disease:

For one thing he doesn't particularly want to go near the man; for another he doesn't care much about his welfare. It would be another thing if Sampe asked for help. Then of course he would do what he could.

Medicines from Oils

The most secretive realm of medical knowledge is the domain of oils: *sakang, sangka', kunti, jang,* and *jayau,* which are essences preserved in coconut oil (*inyak unjer*). They are not physically ingested but magically "fly" into the body of the victim. They each have different purposes, but they all work in the same way. Sakang causes illness or other harm, while sangka' (or *sangga*) is the antidote to a certain sakang. Kunti is a kind of sakang used to protect property, and jang is intended specifically for killing people. Jayau is used to seduce the opposite sex.

The formulas suspended in oil are mysterious and, as far as I can ascertain, are unknown to the Taman. Furthermore, the exact composition appears to be of little interest to the Taman, who receive the charms and medicines already prepared and suspended in oil. The Taman must use the oils according to correct procedures, and may duplicate them as needed. It may be conjectured that the original poisons are similar to those described by Jamuh (1960: 464) for coastal Sarawak, which are reported to contain both plant and animal products, as well as powdered glass, suspended in coconut oil (cf. Gimlette 1971).[4] Any of these oil-based medicines may be reproduced by dipping a cotton swab into a bottle of medicine to absorb the base, placing the swab in a new bottle, and adding oil. (Empty eucalyptus oil containers are commonly used for this purpose.) Thus, in principle, the life of such medicines can be extended indefinitely.

One motive for collecting these esoteric medicines is the power with which they are associated (cf. Helms 1988); the high prices are an indication that the medicines are highly valued. Some frequent observations about the medicines were that they were not available through ordinary means and that not just anyone could obtain them.

Poisoning as a Cause of Illness[5]

The Taman are constantly on guard against black magic such as poisoning and spells. Although their primary fear is that they will be poisoned on a journey away from home, they are also concerned that another Taman who may feel shunned or rejected may want to poison them. For example, if a person asks for something and is rebuffed, that person may feel humiliated; instead of admitting anger, he or she will keep it inside and take revenge on the other with poisons or spells. Given the awkwardness surrounding the refusal of food or drink related to *kempunan* beliefs (see Chapter 4), this widespread suspicion of poisoning is noteworthy, since a guest's failure to receive food or drink is insulting, as it suggests fear of the host.

I was cautioned about the existence of these practices during my stay among the Taman. For example, I was warned not to travel to a certain village because many of the inhabitants possessed poison and might try to put it in my coffee or food. On another occasion, a man told me, "People here have lots of poisons, kuntis, and so forth. If you are given a poison and you know it, give it back. If you don't know, and eat it, you die."

According to informants, the symptoms of poisoning are yellowing of the eyes, mouth, fingernails, or skin; blood in body exuviae (urine, feces, sputum, mucus, sweat, or vomit); blindness; deafness; or paralysis. But depending on the circumstances poison may be the suspected cause of swelling, boils, or any other illness. In one case a man was forced to cancel his plan to travel to Sarawak with a group of companions because he had contracted malaria. Several informants told me it was a case of poisoning. "Poison works like that," said one, "getting worse and worse, taking a year to be noticed if it isn't treated on time." On the other hand another informant said that the suddenness of the disease was a sign that it was a result of poisoning. All informants agreed that poisoning can lead to sudden death if not cured, so the fact that illness lingers is sometimes seen as evidence that an ailment is not from poisoning. They also said that such illnesses were exceedingly difficult to cure.

To Kill a Thief: Kunti

Kunti (also called *munti* or *punti*) is a protective charm consisting of a decoction from roots preserved in oil. It is hidden to protect property, and anyone who trespasses or steals the property suffers weakness, inflammation, or other illnesses characteristic of poisoning. The victim of kunti might die, but unlike poison (jang) it is set up only to protect property and not to kill. But for practical purposes kunti and jang are the same. Some kinds of kunti are *kunti api,* resulting in inflammation; *kunti bajong,* resulting in the victim's leg shriveling up and possibly breaking off; and *kunti pantak* (piercing kunti), causing blindness.

Most informants claimed to know nothing about kunti, saying they are a sin or that they could backfire. In most of the villages I studied, I was unable to get much reliable data on kunti because such devices were said to be unknown. No one admitted to firsthand knowledge of them, and their use was held in contempt. One man said, "People who set up kuntis are no good, they don't have a good attitude. They're dangerous, and people ought to keep a distance from them." The following statement from a village headman is typical:

> I have no experience with *kuntis,* etc. because if you use them wrong they come back to you. I have not used antidotes that combat or protect against poisoning because they are made from the same base as the poison itself. If in a specific instance I had to be treated for poisoning I would make an effort [to find a person who has an antidote], but I don't know who has it.

Antidotes: Sangka'

A number of men owned little bottles of oil that had colored thread tied around their necks. The bottles were kept either hanging from nails on the walls in their houses or in more secretive places. A Taman named Pulok had a kit containing seven medicinal oils, two of which could be used as poisons, and five love medicines. (See Bernstein 1993b for a complete description.)

Among the medicines in the kit was *sangga racun* (antidote to poison). Explaining the medicine, Pulok said, "If you go for a walk, you rub a bit on your chest so you can't be poisoned." The medicine is used to protect against or treat illnesses from poisoning, as indicated by blood in the person's sweat or vomitus. Pulok had obtained it three years previously in Melawi from a Malay, in exchange for a strip of cloth. He uses it whenever he walks and takes it with him wherever he goes.

Another of Pulok's oils was *sakang dilangkah* ("stepped-on" sakang), capable of causing harm as well as treating harm from poisoning. The oil is rubbed on property; if a person attempts to steal the property, his or her body swells up. Sakang dilangkah can also be rubbed on a doorpost in order to prevent a thief from entering. The oil can be used as *sakang kunti,* but if a needle is added to the container, it can cause death. Although this is not allowed, as it would constitute murder, Pulok commented, "That's okay if you really do want to kill the person." This substance is also the only medicine effective in treating illness caused by this charm, as well as a variety of swellings not caused by magic. He had used it both to protect himself from poisoning and to cure a Taman man who had swelling in different parts of his body. According to Pulok, anyone treated with this oil must pay Rp 5,000 for the treatment, but in this case the man paid an equivalent amount by offering him a chicken and a knife in addition to Rp 2,000 in cash.

Several other Taman people whom I interviewed owned similar medicines. All said they had bought them, obtained them in exchange, or inherited them. One man said he had been given them by guests passing through. A woman showed me a bottle of antidote to poison she and her husband had bought in Mandai in 1982 for Rp 30,000 (at the time more than US$50). Inside the bottle were a sewing needle, some red thread, and green coconut oil. Anyone who brings poison near it starts to shake and is soon forced to leave. The medicine is rubbed on the body, and one can travel anywhere without fear of being poisoned. They keep another bottle of the same medicine in a little plastic bag tied behind a post inside the front door to protect their house from theft.

Another informant had three medicines, each obtained in different places. One of these, *sangga tapang,* was intended "to make someone nervous, so that if someone says something it will not come to pass." The second was *sakang seribu,* "antidote for a thousand poisons," used to treat all ailments except malaria. The third was a pair of antidotes working together as "husband" and "wife" to cause illness from poisoning or kunti to return to its source. He has never mentioned his possession of these medicines to his fellow Taman villagers.

The sangka' for kunti is derived from the same plant as the harmful kunti itself. The poison is made from the western side of the plant (the side of the setting sun), and the antidote is made from the eastern side (the side of the rising sun).

A woman showed me a bottle containing the sangka' for kunti bajong, in which there were also sewing needles. She said that each person who uses this medicine must place a needle into the bottle as "food" for the medicine so that the kunti will not "eat" him or her. She came to acquire this sangka', she said, when her husband had owned a coffee grove that was frequently raided by thieves. Some people from Mandai came through the area to sell clothes and other goods, and her husband, who was their host, told them of their losses. The men took pity on her husband and gave him a kunti; therefore, he was also given the antidote. According to her, when the husband moved to Sarawak, he sold the kunti, leaving only the antidote with his wife.

Despite the disincentives to admit to ownership of these medicines, people who have effective medicines become known through informal conversation, and ailing people travel from other villages to seek their medication. One man charged for treatment Rp 10,000 plus a chicken, a knife, one gantang of rice, and a meter of white cloth.

It is hazardous to use a medicine illicitly, without knowing its specifications, because each medicine is associated with certain prohibitions on food or drink. The danger of consuming prohibited food is that, if the illness returns, the medicine will be unable to cure it. It is recognized that people disobey these prohibitions because of an appetite for the forbidden foods. I was told about such a case in which a person was given a list of prohibited foods. He disregarded the proscription, and was dead in two days.

A Case of Kunti and Its Treatment

The case of Rasid, a twenty-year-old man, provides a good illustration of the way kunti is treated by the Taman. Rasid returned to his village with a severely swollen leg after working as a lumberjack in a distant part of the district. He had been working as part of a group of about fifteen young men when he and a Kayan companion were affected—he on the leg and the other man in the groin. They knew of no natural explanation (such as an insect bite) for the malady. A healer in the vicinity discovered that the illness originated from their trespassing on other people's property with the intention of cutting down trees; the grounds had been protected by an oil, kunti bajong, which had caused the swelling. The healer treated them with leaves, roots, dirt, an ants' nest, and water in which rice had been rinsed. Feeling somewhat better, and realizing that no one there could treat them, they returned home. Those closely connected with the young man and familiar with his circumstances said that if he did not get well, he would have to return to the spot where he had been afflicted and appeal for help from the owner of the land (whom he had sought unsuccessfully) on which he had trespassed.

The illness worsened again, and a Kalis man who lived in a neighboring Taman village was brought in to treat him. He expressed optimism about Rasid's prognosis and said that, while he would try to help, he could not promise success. "If the medicine does not work for him," he said, "the patient can be treated by someone else." If his condition worsened, it would not be his fault.

His treatment consisted of the administration of medicines from two vials, both containing swabs of cotton submerged in coconut oil, and said to work together as "husband and wife," as "antidotes for a thousand poisons" (sakang seribu). It was apparent that, apart from possessing these medicines and being able to administer them, he did not claim to be, nor could he be considered, a healer. The Kalis man said that he had inherited these medicines from his father and that no one outside his line of descent could use them. He did not know the origin of the medicines or who first made them, but he said his grandfather had given them to him and taught him how to use them. He had taught him to "feed" each of the two medicines a bit of ground metal every month, so that they would not die of hunger, and coconut oil, so that they would not dry out.

Before going to Rasid's home, he performed a test: He dipped a "needle" (a sliver of nipa palm leaf on which incense fumes have settled) into the "male" bottle; if drops fell off, the patient would get well. If not, he would dip the needle into the "female" bottle. If no drops fell off this needle either, it meant the medicine would not work. If that had in fact happened, he would have refused to treat Rasid.

To treat Rasid, the Kalis man dipped the nipa leaf into the male bottle and rubbed it on his own hands three times. He did the same with the medicine in the female bottle. Then seven times he rubbed the medicine from his hands onto the bad leg of the patient with a downward motion, saying, "You, who are sick, must get well. Struck by bajong, struck by punti, this is your medicine. The disease is leaving your body like a shirt being taken off." As he tenderly stroked the oil on Rasid's bad leg, he warned him that it could cause extreme pain or burning, because such illnesses usually "combat" the medicine as it enters the body and breaks down the disease. In one hour, he applied the medicine about ten times. Before leaving, he mixed cooking oil given to him by Rasid's mother with medicine from both the male and female bottles, putting the mixture into a new bottle. This medicine was to be used by the patient over the coming days as necessary.

Treatment with the medicine entailed several prohibitions of particular foods and work. The food prohibitions applied to, among other things, papaya, watermelon, freshwater fish, and ground chilies. These prohibitions are supposed to be observed all the patient's life to prevent the illness from returning in an incurable form. The prohibition of work for one month was a guideline and needed to be observed only until the patient felt well. (While some food prohibitions may be dropped depending on the patient's recovery, the transgression of others is thought to bring on a relapse.)

The Kalis man described the payment for the treatment as a *pelias*: to protect him from the ancestors, so the illness he treated might not enter his own body.[6] Payment included a gantang of rice, a 90-centimeter strip (*lerang*) of blue cloth, a knife (*parang*), a sewing needle, a glass bowl, thread, and Rp 1,000 in cash—"as much as the family can afford to spare."

Erotic Pharmacology: Jayau

Other magical oils used by the Taman are those called jayau, intended to cause someone to fall in love with the person using it. Unlike the oil-based antidotes to poisons, this "erotic pharmacology" (Winkler 1990: 79) seems to be at least partly indigenous, since certain ingredients are traced to known mythologized topography. The best-known jayau base is *buluh merindu* (longing bamboo). The Taman believe that buluh merindu grows in the vicinity of Bukit Tilung in Mandai Subdistrict, the land of the dead (see Chapter 4).[7]

Buluh merindu is not the only love medicine known to the Taman. Harrisson (1965: 270–271) mentions a stone that came into being as the result of the petrification of an incestuous couple; it is preserved in oil, and "today's charm is any fungus or waste collected from the *breasts* of the petrification" (emphasis in the original). (People are warned not to use such waste from the "private parts" of the stone, at the risk of the user's becoming oversexed.) To use this charm, a person rubs it on his or her own face, saying, "So and so, you must love me."

One man showed me three bottles containing jayau, telling me that it was "woman medicine" (that is, medicine to charm a woman). He explained, "You give it to a girl if she doesn't want you." The bottles each contain fishing hooks, "gifts" to the medicine. "If not given, the medicine cannot live," he said.

A number of married men owned these medicines, saying they had bought them in Mandai from Kalis people. The informant just mentioned said that many people buy these to take with them to Malaysia, where they use them on women.[8] Pulok, a 65-year-old Taman man, not only had five jayau ("star oil," "taro oil," "woman sweetener," "water buffalo oil," and "sweetener") but also possessed a charm (purportedly a squirrel's penis inserted through a piece of wood) supposed to make a man's erection last all night.

As with the other oil-based charms, and probably more so, there is a profit motive in collecting these jayau. My informants agreed that many people collect these medicines with the intention of selling them at a profit, and that a tidy profit could in fact be made from these oils. The most likely opportunities for using these oils—and acquiring them—occur during travels, when men are not bound by their obligations at home. Another possible use is for youthful couples who love each other but whose parents forbid their marriage. The frustrated boy may give the medicine to his girlfriend to make her disobey her parents. About these oils, Pulok said:

> No one may borrow them. Anyone wanting to use them must buy them. People around here don't know anything about how they are made. They cannot be given as gifts. Also, they are not a game. You can only use them on your own wife, or to get a wife if you are divorced or widowed. If you already have a wife you may not use it. People around here *very* often use these devices to get wives.

Clearly, it is dangerous to use jayau for adulterous purposes, considering the strict penalties on sexual misbehavior in Taman society (see Chapter 2). While many people apparently put much credence in these charms, one man said he did not believe in love magic because love is from destiny or fate (*kebetulan*), from God. Jayau, he said, can make a dead person come to life and kill a living person. Therefore, he reasoned, anyone experienced with these oils would not want to use them but would throw them away. Two teenagers whom I interviewed said they were afraid of love medicine—they were not yet ready for marriage, and the use of these oils would inevitably lead to that. The point that my informants made clear is that with jayau, as with other oils, anyone who wants to use them is free to do so but must be prepared to accept the consequences of their effectiveness.

Malay Healers and Their Cures

Even in the most distant Taman villages, some 12 miles (20 kilometers) from Putussibau, Malay healers, known as dukuns, play an important role.[9] Several highly regarded dukuns, and a larger number of less well-known occasional practitioners, reside in villages in the outskirts of Putussibau. None of them live within the boundaries of Putussibau itself, a fact probably explainable by both the higher real estate values there and the greater "folk" ambience of the outlying Malay villages. Some dukuns have connections of friendship or kinship with the Taman people; one even owns a house in a Taman village. Taman people may consult Malay dukuns when in town or make a special visit to a dukun to get herbal medications to take home to sick family members. Certain illnesses are said to be curable only by dukuns, among them *karawan bawi* (epilepsy; see Chapter 4) and *karoranan* (a fish bone or fruit pit caught in the throat).

Dukuns attribute most illnesses to wind and ghosts, but they do not favor any particular explanation of illness. Many dukuns are adept at diagnosing and countering spells and charms, and most are also proficient at using herbal remedies for treating illnesses not attributed to any external intentional agent, spirit or human.

The word "healer" does not adequately convey the versatility of skills attributed to the dukun, who would perhaps better be described as a wizard (cf. Winstedt 1951). The dukun not only cures illness but divines fortunes and can solve problems by either casting or breaking a spell. If property has been lost, the dukun may cause it to return, or he may use his proficiency to identify and punish the thief. A dukun's services may be solicited to make a protective amulet containing a Koranic verse for a newborn baby. Although the Taman are mainly Christianized, these amulets are routinely commissioned by them. Malay healing also focuses on sexual problems. While issues of male potency and female frigidity are addressed, charms and therapies concentrate at least as much on such matters as jealousy, fidelity, and compatibility (including simultaneous orgasm). A dukun's spell can make a person love or hate another person.

Mystical Knowledge

Although most dukuns claimed that the basis of their practice was inherited tradition and divine scripture, their methods of healing varied substantially. They all used some combination of spells, charms, and herbal medicaments, but the basis of their practice, they said, was *ilmu*. *Ilmu* is an Arabic-derived Malay-Indonesian word, the standard meaning of which is "knowledge" or "science"; however, in the context of Malay medicine it refers to "mystical knowledge."

The source and authority of knowledge in Malay medicine is attributed to the Koran. Spoken and written charms and blessings from this and other sacred writings are used in Malay healing. Blessings are intoned over medicines, and blessed water is also thought to possess curative powers.

Explaining the meaning of ilmu as "healing power," a dukun named Rachman said, "My ilmu is not to glorify myself, not for self-esteem or self-aggrandizement. I don't treat people before the other dukun, but after. I am the last resort."

Another dukun, Ali, said he uses "nothing but Indonesian ilmu," inherited knowledge from past generations. He used the term *ilmu jiwa* to refer to the phrenological reading or measurement of bodily characteristics he performs. (In standard Indonesian, this term means "psychology"—literally "soul science.") He diagnoses illness by feeling under the eyes, ears, and mouth to determine whether a person has been sickened by the work of another. Ali said he had acquired ilmu from his own experiences regarding people's facial complexions, as well as from a book written in Arabic that he had memorized.

People who possess ilmu are known for their ability to make lost objects return. For example, one dukun said he could make a person who had robbed someone feel heat in his stomach until he could no longer tolerate the pain and would be forced to return the object. Another dukun said he could make any stolen object return, except a cow that had already been slaughtered and eaten; his charm to bring the cow back would cause innocent people to die. He added that what made the lost object return was people's fear of his ilmu.

This ilmu derives ostensibly from the Koran, and so can be learned by anyone inclined to do so. A number of books have been printed about charms, amulets, and cures and are sold in stalls at the Putussibau market. The system, known as *mujarrobat* (literally "effective medicine"), is a syncretic mixture of scriptural Islam, Arabian folklore, and Malay magic. It is part of a larger set of prayers and talismans to cure illness or solve problems, information about the meanings of dreams, and astrology and numerology. Several cures are for sexual problems. For example, men who must leave their wives for long periods are advised to extract several cc's of their blood, put it in a bottle, and bury it for forty days, then mix the blood with their semen. This mixture is to be put into the woman's food or drink to insure her faithful love. Other charms and spells—often called "medicines"—are intended to catch thieves, to prevent a house from burning down, to become wealthy, and to prevent pests from eating crops (*Mujarrobat Madiinatual Asroor* 1980). Dukuns often compile their own treatises in notebooks.

The Taman have incorporated many of the Malays' practices, such as the pusau described earlier, and a number of them have sought to learn this ilmu. The Malay dukun Rachman said that a Taman balien once studied under him for several days. Another Taman man who also studied under this healer had learned several magical sayings to cure disease. This man's son had also studied with Rachman and recorded in a notebook a number of his spells. Yet another Taman man—Pulok, a nominal Protestant—showed me some Arabic script books he had bought in Malaysia (one of which he claimed dated from the year 92) that contained magical incantations.

Ilmu can obviously be put to harmful purposes in certain hands. It can be used to cause illness, death, or misfortune, through spells or charms. It is thought that the ghosts of people who attained an overabundance of ilmu are dangerous. In spite of the possibility that they may possess a dangerous knowledge of black magic, the dukuns consider their role to be that of one who helps people by curing them, through the permission of God. The well-established dukuns are not feared by either townspeople or villagers, and it is recognized that they have no interest in the malicious use of their powers. People of many religions, ethnic groups, and social strata seek their services, sometimes traveling from relatively distant regions to consult them. Nevertheless, several dukuns undoubtedly cultivate an aura of mystery.

Louis Golomb (1985: 195) notes that healing specialists from ethnic minorities in both Thailand and Malaysia tend to be sought mostly for those "services requiring confidentiality but not intimacy." If a surreptitious relationship with a magical healer is desired, an outsider is probably preferable to a member of one's own group. Golomb suggests, however, that people patronize healers outside their own group mainly when an illicit service is sought, such as the casting or countering of a spell; for the cure of illness, outsiders are consulted only as a last resort. My data contradict this finding; I commonly observed Taman and other non-Malay patients being treated by Malay healers.

The Dukun's Treatments and Medicines

The esoteric knowledge possessed by dukuns is used straightforwardly; incantations are taught to any clients who care to learn them. However, dukuns use not only ilmu but also special medicines, purported to be panaceas or antidotes to a thousand poisons. They may also have vials containing other special oils, such as "star oil" or "lightning oil," which are considered extremely rare and difficult to store. Dukuns use special techniques or paraphernalia such as feathers in applying these oils, although some medicines are ingested by patients. The reputation of the dukun stems in part from the potency of his medicines. Like ilmu, these oils are cloaked in mystery. As one dukun said, his medicine was inherited and could not be manufactured. It is possible, however, to replenish supplies of these medicines by adding cooking oil to the base. Some dukuns also use a large number of medicinal plants that they usually growing in their gardens. Some of the materials they use are exotic to the Putussibau area. One dukun uses wax in some of his therapies and frogs' blood in others.

Malay medicine is characterized by a distinct emphasis on cure-alls. Dukuns vary in their emphasis on herbalism, amulets, and charms or spells. Many use special paraphernalia for which unique properties are claimed. One dukun, Ali, has a broken pair of scissors that he claimed to have made himself, on instructions from God. He uses the scissors sometimes by themselves and sometimes with two magnets. For headaches, he rolls the scissors in the patient's hair. He also uses the scissors to treat madness, impotence, and muteness. He explains: "If the person isn't sick there's no current. If the pain is on the right side of the back I place the scissors between the toes on the right side, and vice versa. If a person is made sick from within, by worrying too much or thinking too hard, it can't be treated." Rachman, another dukun, possessed a large assortment of paraphernalia, including two charms—one a talisman called Lam Awal that he said was 1,468 years old[10] and claimed contained scripture about the prophets, and the other containing a string and a bit of deer horn—and a bottle of magical star oil (*minyak bintang*) to rid the patient of illnesses caused by "man-made winds." He uses these for a treatment called *tepas*.

In this treatment the patient sits on a mat while Rachman spreads a sheet over his body. He rubs the two amulets over the patient's body while reciting the following blessing: "*Assalamualaikum Sih Lukman ul-Hakim. Bukan kuasaku, kuasa Allah.*"[11] Rachman then strokes the amulets on the patient, then brushes the patient off. The first blessing is followed by the "king blessing," uttered three times: *Bismillah hiri-hiri, Permata datin permata jati.*"[12] The patient stands up and brushes herself or himself off. The dukun taps the dirt from the mat into a bowl of water. He covers the patient again with a sheet, brushes the patient with one amulet in his right hand, then uses the other amulet, which he also places in his right hand. Then he dips a feather in star oil, removes the sheet, and waves the feather over the patient for a few seconds, barely touching the patient's body. The dirt is shaken into the bowl, the mat is rolled up, and then Rachman instructs the patient to spit in the bowl. Rachman writes the "Arabic" character Robmin (see Figure 3.1) in the water with a knife.[13] Rachman explains that when the dirt (bearing the disease) falls in the bowl, it is still alive, and the figure Robmin is drawn "so the disease will die." The water is then thrown out. The dukun pours a glass of water from a pitcher, says a blessing over it, and blows on it. Again he

Figure 3.1 Robmin. This character is "written" with a knife in a bowl of water "so the disease will die." Enlargement of a drawing by Rachman.

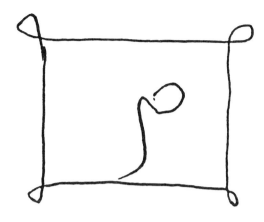

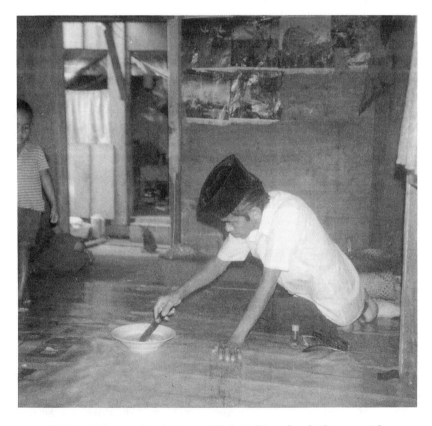

Rachman draws the character "Robmin" in a bowl of water with a knife to kill the disease that has been taken out of the patient's body.

says the blessing and blows on it. The water is given to the patient, who drinks it.[14]

This was not Rachman's only therapy, but he performed it on every patient who came to him. He did so unceremoniously, but with a fine clinical bearing. Once, for example, he looked into the bowl in which the disease had supposedly been shaken out and chuckled, saying, "A lot came out." He asks patients how they feel and whether they have experienced any change in their symptoms, and he touches them to find where it hurts. He offers diagnoses in a manner that is authoritative and assuring. He names the foods that must be avoided and prepares herbal medicines for patients to take home with them. He knows a variety of medicines as well as spells and counterspells and handles each case on its clinical features. However, his medicine is the medicine of the paradoxical. As he says, his specialty is curing illnesses that have no medicine.

Many of these dukuns can speak at length and with considerable erudition about their medicines and the characteristics of diseases. Hassan, who provided me with a typewritten list of spells, also contributed a similar list of village illnesses that he said were incurable by government medicine. In a primarily oral folk society these men are specialists knowledgeable of the mystical powers of written words. (See Sweeney 1987.)

Dukuns use a number of ingredients and techniques in their medicines. Their herbal pharmacopoeia includes a range of flowers, leaves, herbs, woods, vines, and barks. Rachman, for example, relied heavily in his therapy on turmeric and yellow ginger (*Curcuma xanthorrhiza*), while another dukun I studied was partial to the leaves of a plant called *juaran* (Rubiaceae). Dukuns also use eggs or water, over which they recite spells or blessings, and lime, often mixed with an herb such as turmeric, painted on the patient's body.

Besides varying in their specific techniques, there is considerable specialization in the focus of the dukun's practices: Some may concentrate on children's illnesses, while others say they can treat anyone but children; some plead an inability to cure illness caused by poisoning or sorcery, while others specialize in just such illnesses. Other dukuns specialize not in curing illness but in the recovery of lost objects. The dukuns consider their cures to be incompatible with the healing ceremonies of Taman and other Dayak shamans.

While the dukun may have many specific cures, he is above all a generalist. Rachman's claim that he specializes in curing those illnesses for which there is no medicine is perspicacious. Dukuns lack biomedical insight into standard diagnostic features of disease.

Although the dukun's healing technique starts from a simple theoretical structure, in practice, it often manifests itself as a hodgepodge of heterogeneous practices to solve a large range of problems. The dukun's craft can well be compared to what Claude Lévi-Strauss called *bricolage*: "a logic

whose terms consist of odds and ends left over from psychological processes" (1966: 35). In Malay medicine, as in bricolage, all manner of complaints
and illnesses are classified and treated using some combination of a small
number of charms and herbal medications dukuns have at their disposal.

Case Studies

Rachman.   Pak Rachman is an extremely popular healer and there are usually people in his house either being treated or waiting for him. He seems to
be especially favored by Taman villagers.

Born in Bunut (a small town downstream of Putussibau) in 1930,
Rachman developed a lung ailment that no dukun could heal and stayed in
the hospital in Putussibau for four months. With the help of God he got well.
In a dream he saw his parents, who taught him a sacred verse: "Peace unto
you, Sheikh Lukman ul-Hakim. Not my power, but the power of Allah."
After that dream, whenever he ate he would recite this. In ten days he was
out of the hospital. Since then he has never been ill. After this incident a
sacred book was given to him within which he found the same phrase. This
experience confirmed for him his vocation as a divinely inspired healer.

Rachman says he studies medicine from books and he must practice an
incantation ten times before he can commit it to memory. His incantations
(*tawar*) originated with his ancestors in Bunut, "in the days before there was
religion." They refer to Mount Reban and the Badi Sea, the origin of all disease. He gets some prayers from a book, *Mujarrobat Melayu Lengkap*
(*Complete Malay Medicine*), but he has also compiled charms, cures, and
mystical information in notebooks of his own, which he consults from time
to time. Along with his use of other medicines, he intones blessings over
water, red onions, or eggs. Among his incantations are one for a woman who
wants beautiful long hair, one to cure snake bites, and one to make a person
become so ugly that no one will want to look at him or her. Rachman claims
he can cast pain-inducing spells over people; however, he says his magic
cannot kill anyone.

Rachman supports himself solely on his income as a healer. He claims
not to have any other employment because he "doesn't know how to work."
He accepts whatever people give him and does not demand a set fee. This
has resulted in some patients apparently taking advantage of his good
nature. Often people promise to pay him but never do, or a family has a
patient stay at his house for extended periods of time without even providing food. He complains that people from the villages forget their promises
to him after they have been cured but adds that other people's generosity
makes up for that. He has a forgiving attitude to the nonpayers.

Rachman is reputed to be a particularly versatile healer. The only thing
he admits he is unable to cure is illness caused by poisoning. Rachman says

he can also tell if he is unable to cure a patient based on the position of the sun or the color of the patient's clothing. He possesses scores of remedies, among them a cure for najam (chest pains): crushed *mentemu* (*Curcuma xanthorrhiza*) mixed with egg, juaran leaf, and water, stroked on the body. He has cures for headache, childhood diseases, toothache, and many other ailments. As he himself says, his specialty is treating illness and not determining the cause. On occasion he or his wife goes to Bunut to obtain certain medicinal roots and woods that are unavailable in the Putussibau vicinity, but he grows in his garden most of the herbs he usually needs.

Hassan.   Hassan, born in Putussibau in 1940, is a mysterious man who has a regular job and is often called away for reasons he will not elaborate. In his healing work he relies on the theories of his great-grandfather, a learned man who had studied the holy scriptures from the ages of thirty-eight to sixty-two. Hassan was very close to him, and slept under the same mosquito net with him. His great-grandfather wrote out everything in Arabic script. It took Hassan six months to learn it by heart. After the instruction was complete, Hassan was ceremonially bathed, and announced that he intended to emulate his great-grandfather by becoming a dukun.

Hassan specializes in the return of lost objects, although he performs a range of medicinal cures as well. His main medicines are *jimat*s (amulets) and juaran leaves. His amulets are different from Rachman's, and unlike Rachman, he uses neither eggs nor mentemu in his medicine, nor does he use tepas.[15]

Ali.   Ali was born in 1929 in Putussibau. He attended school for three years, was married when he was 16, and became a farmer. When he was young, he learned Arabic, and when he was 25 he became a dukun. His medicine is "inherited" and cannot be made. He says that he cannot make a living being a dukun but only does it to help people. He charges Rp.5,000 or its equivalent in rice to cure a person. In an interview he claimed that in the previous month sixty people had come to him for treatment. He is often wild and bedraggled of appearance, and in his manner he seems to cultivate a reputation of being involved with the supernatural. A competing dukun said of him that "he is an expert at flying, and also at sinning." Another colleague said that Ali wore the same clothes every day because they protect his body so powerfully that bullets cannot penetrate.

Ali, who treats patients primarily with an oil, differentiates completely between treatment for adults and children and says that he cannot treat children.

Relationship to Competing Systems of Healing

Malay dukuns see themselves fitting into the pluralistic medical system and working in cooperation with doctors and hospitals. They claim that doctors ask them to help cure those patients they are unable to cure themselves. One dukun said that he would go to the hospital to care for patients: "For injections, doctors and nurses take charge, and for traditional treatment they leave it in my hands." Asked about this claim, a doctor in Putussibau said that the families of patients often ask if they may call in folk healers and that the doctors allow it. These dukuns consider their work to be incompatible with that of Taman and other Dayak shamans. Rachman, for example, disparages the work of the shamans as collaboration with the Devil, in contrast to his own cures, which are effective because of God's mercy. He claims that the blessings he uses scare away the spirits that are effective in the shaman's therapy. He never attends balien or other shamanistic ceremonies, saying that Islamic law forbids him from being present at such heathen practices. Furthermore, he says, a shaman who saw him at such a ceremony would be unable to catch the patient's soul. Significantly, he does not deny that the balien can be effective in treating the illnesses of some patients.

Omar, another dukun, differentiates his healing practice from that of Mujarrobat dukuns such as Rachman, as well as from that of the Taman balien. He says his healing is facilitated by the *jin* (spirits of the earth), while that of the balien is facilitated by other spirits he calls *dewa* (gods), which inhabit the sky. He believes his cures, in which he uses seven kinds of flowers and two kinds of leaves, are magical. He says that whereas the mujarrobat dukun looks in the book to see what plants to use, the jin dukun speaks directly to the jin. "Jin healing is indeed strange," Omar said. "Sometimes it doesn't make sense, but the patient can be cured."

"Government Medicine"

Government medicine is thought to cure only those diseases originating within the body—"diseases of condition," as one informant put it. The Taman people I studied were quite dissatisfied with the quality of medical care provided by the government.

The main hospital in Putussibau is unsanitary and in disrepair. My informants said that it had formerly been run by the Catholic Church and had declined in quality after the government took it over. Two doctors based in Putussibau service the entire subdistrict. Both doctors work from their offices at home and serve at the clinic. The army base in Putussibau (far from the center of town and best reached by bicycle or motorcycle) has its own clinic with its own staff. Medicines are scarce, and anything out of the ordinary is unavailable. A few people specialize in making false teeth. Pharmacies, which with few exceptions are operated by Chinese, specialize in patent medicines. Many people in the Putussibau area who need serious medical attention prefer, if money and circumstances allow it, to travel to distant cities in Kalimantan or Sarawak, or even to Jakarta.

The government has built Public Health Centers (*Puskesmas*) in three villages and assigned *mantris* (medical aides or male nurses) from Sintang to the centers in Melapi and Siut. A Public Health Center was also built in Sibau Hilir, but the mantri assigned to that village refused to move in unless the cattle were fenced in to prevent them from freely roaming the village. This was accomplished, but the government never sent him back, and the building—the only one with glass windows in the entire village—was vacant and deteriorating during my stay.

Provisions for the centers lag far behind requisitions; few kinds of medicines are available, and syringes must be reused. The population generally distrusts the dressers, suspecting them of administering adulterated and stale medicine to boost profits. The Taman also believe that their syringes are dirty and cause infection.

It is widely believed that medicine from abroad, in contrast to Indonesian-manufactured medicine, is effective. One man said that during the Dutch age a sick person could get better after only one injection, but that nowadays even three or four injections may not be enough.

These doubts about government medicine are put aside in times of illness, when the Taman seek pharmaceutical remedies whenever possible. However, it appears that the Taman people frequently fail to comply with doctors' instructions to continue using medicines. Many people own stocks of medicines that they stopped taking after a day, having decided that they were not fit for their illness.

Conclusion

This chapter has described a range of medicinal cures, from the most commonplace to esoteric medicines that require specific procedures and are socially consequential. The Taman see medicine as a vital essence that must be fed, is adversarial in nature, can cause harm as well as good, and can backfire on its owner if not treated correctly.

The high prices claimed for medicines to which access is limited suggest that they are highly valued. People acquire knowledge of medicines on sojourns outside Taman society. Returning to their villages, people guard their knowledge as a special possession that should not be freely dispensed. Older men have the most knowledge (and biggest collections) of medicines, while women rarely possess any unless they have traveled. The accumulation of these medicines is a route to a kind of esoteric power (cf. Helms 1988: 111–130). Other medicines are personal—gifts from spirits encountered in dreams. In either case, possession of medicine is never made public; rather, a person wanting to use another's medicine must make a private request, and payment is usually required. Finally, these medicines are considered dangerous, and it is insinuated that those who collect them may have evil motives. In contrast to the balien, who is obliged to treat (for payment) any person requesting healing, those who treat people informally with these medicines or charms may deny treatment by concealing their powers.

This attitude toward exotic medicines among the Taman has resulted in the sensitization of discourse on more common medicines. The extreme reluctance to display medicines or publicize ownership of them is striking. Ownership of certain medicinal oils confers powers not in keeping with social norms. Pressure from neighbors to dispense medicine generously on demand is considered onerous, and the Taman prefer to avoid these demands through concealment. This preference for concealment and secrecy is reinforced by the occult and mystified status of the dukun.

Notes

1. On the concept of a "profession" of medicine, see Chapter 7.
2. A reader has suggested that the notion that ownership implies an obligation to share is perhaps related to the requirements surrounding *kempunan* (see Chapter 4). This is an intriguing possibility, but I am not convinced of its validity. No informants mentioned such an explanation. Kempunan is caused by failing to partake in the consumption of something another person is also consuming, to satisfy an urge or to complete an action. While an ethos of sharing and reciprocity may underlie kempunan beliefs and practices, people are not expected to share whatever they have, nor do they have a right to claim another person's property.
3. I was unable to collect a specimen.
4. From the publications of Jamuh and Gimlette it appears that many of these poisons are effective. It is interesting to note, in this connection, that apart from a few regulations concerning *jimats* (see below) and the teaching of magic knowledge and skills, "the problem of magic, sorcery, and witchcraft is, from the legalistic perspective, nonexistent in Indonesian law" (Slaats and Portier 1993: 138).
5. This category corresponds to "sorcery." There is no concept of a witch, that is, a member of human society (though perhaps not truly a human being) who is inherently capable of causing illness or other misfortune.
6. "This is probably from the Malay *perkeras* (or *pekras* or *kras*) meaning 'hand' but used to refer to the required ritual payment to a curer or other specialist" (Robert Winzeler, personal communication).
7. Harrisson (1965: 318) provides a more exact location: "all over the range of hills of Bukit Sunan, Bukit Liang Karang, and Bukit Apo Andan in the upper Kalis river." He calls the bamboo *buluh pengerindu,* which has a synonymous meaning to *buluh merindu,* which he also mentions. Stories about buluh merindu are found throughout Indonesia, and it is mentioned in traditional verse (Amin Sweeney, personal communication), though presumably without reference to Bukit Tilung.
8. I have no data on women's use of jayau. Malay healers have many charms available for women who want to make their husbands faithful to them, but the use of instrumental seduction magic seems to be a masculine preoccupation. Of course, it is also possible that there exist whole realms of women's esoteric knowledge and practices that are resistant to the investigations of a male ethnographer. Aside from occult issues, such information, which may be confided to a trusted member of one's own sex, would be a betrayal of the interests of one's sex if given to the opposite sex. Tsing (1993: 215–228) provides narrative accounts of several Dayak women who had love affairs with foreign men. Like my material on love medicine, these narra-

tives were freely given to her. I cannot imagine such information being entrusted to a male anthropologist. As Gregory (1984) has shown, the feminist claim of male bias in social anthropology has been generally overstated; nevertheless, it cannot be denied that gender issues figure in ethnographer-informant relations.

9. Other Malay terms for the folk healer, *bomoh* and *pawang,* were not used, though they were recognized by some of my Malay informants.

10. Probably a reference to the time of the prophet Muhammad.

11. "Peace unto you, Sheikh Lukman ul-Hakim. Not my power, but the power of Allah." Sheikh Lukman ul-Hakim, according to the informant, is "a person who knows the origin of the world." Mohd. Taib bin Osman (1972: 227) writes that most Malay *bomoh*s (dukuns) "ascribe the origin of their office to the legendary figure of Luqman al-hakim."

12. A standard invocation based on the Arabic *Bismillahir rohmanir rohim* ("In the name of Allah the compassionate, the merciful"). The second phrase means, "Your diamond is the true diamond." This "king blessing" is said by Rachman to have a thousand uses.

13. There is no Arabic or Jawi (Arabic-based Malay script) character called Robmin. This character resembles both the Jawi letters *ra* (r) and the unconnected *mim* (m), but Robmin itself is not a word either in Arabic or Malay.

14. There are variations in the tepas method, and a version of it is performed by some Taman healers using *suri* (*Cordyline fruticosa*) leaves instead of amulets.

15. He did, however, mention that the rhizome is an elixir to be drunk by those who have a loss of appetite, weakness of body, and balien's syndrome. This rhizome, called *tantamu* by the Taman, is a necessary part of the balien's armamentarium and in fact is drunk during the initiation ceremony.

4

Explanations of Illness and Their Conceptual Framework

The concepts of illness described in this chapter are part of larger cultural systems and must be understood in the context of a larger set of background premises.[1] These concepts are not entirely specific to the Taman; they are shared to some extent by other peoples throughout the Upper Kapuas and to a lesser extent in other parts of Borneo and beyond. The balien system is only one of the folk healing systems to which the Taman have recourse. Furthermore, there are several templates for comprehending illness that can be summed up in the distinction between the notion that illness is internally caused and the notion that it is externally caused, or sent. The latter concept includes ideas about spirits and ghosts, spells, poisons, and charms.

Among the Taman, the tendency to explain illness as originating outside the body is dominant, though not universal. Not only baliens but other folk-medical specialists and other healers mostly concentrate on the treatment of externally caused illnesses. As a whole, the Taman medical belief system may be described as an "externalizing" one, in Allan Young's (1976b) terms.

> *Externalizing systems* concentrate on making etiological explanations for serious sicknesses. Here, pathogenic agencies are usually purposive and often human or anthropomorphized. Diagnostic interests concentrate on discovering what events could have brought the sick person to the attention of the pathogenic agency . . . in order to identify the responsible category of pathogen, or, even, the responsible individual agent. . . . Often only gross symptomatic distinctions are made, since the intrasomatic links between etiological events and sequences of biophysical signs are not elaborated. (Young 1976b: 148)

While the Taman tend to think of illness as externally caused, they recognize that certain illnesses originate from within a person's own body. Illnesses originating from outside the body cannot be treated with medicines or therapies suited for those originating within the body, and vice versa. For example, diseases originating from the skin cannot be cured by any of the balien's methods. However, if a skin disease is from an external cause, it can be so treated. Actually, this logic works the other way around: If a balien treats and successfully cures a skin disease, that is proof that the pathology was external.

The understanding of illness underlying all balien practices is that it is the result of the action of a spirit being on the human soul. Thus, an explication of the concepts of souls and spirits is central to an explanation of the balien institution. The concept of illness is situated in a framework that looks at illness in the context of the nature of the human soul and what happens to it in dreams and death. Following a discussion of these topics, I describe and analyze specific ideas about how and, equally important, why spirits attack the soul. I then consider explanations of illness as resulting from the wind, spells, and internal causes.

Kinds of Spirits

The spirit world consists of demons (*sai*), ghosts (*antu*), and goblins (jin). The words for ghost and goblin are Malay, and it is unclear whether the Taman have an indigenous concept of a ghost (as opposed to a demon) that is distinct from the Malay concept. A majority of informants considered sai and antu to have the same meaning; they were "unseen beings." The word *jalu* (thing or object) is often used in terms that refer to diseases: *dawawa jalu, dabalas jalu, datorok jalu, dasumpit jalu, jalu tio,* and others. One informant differentiated between antu and sai, saying that antu can be frightened away by people, whereas sai can inflict disease in a person's body. Being invisible, they can attack undetected. Thus, for the Taman there are a plurality of different kinds of spirits. The Taman know that the spirits of their own villages and places, recounted in folklore, are not the only kinds; spirits known to the Muslim Malay and other peoples are also real to the Taman and can affect them. Although Malay concepts of spirits have probably penetrated Taman ideas about spirits to an extent, the Taman concept of spirit (sai or *pamari'an*) is distinct and is the basis of the balien institution.

Baliens are the main authorities on sai, while knowledge about antu is more widely distributed. Only baliens have controlled, extensive, firsthand knowledge of spirits; others usually report knowing very little about them. Most informants said that a nonbalien could not see the sai. (Only one nonbalien informant claimed to have ever directly encountered a sai. He said that they look like animals such as mousedeer, bears, or orangutans, among others, and added that many people have seen them.)

A whole world of spirits unseen by ordinary people is visible to the balien. I was occasionally told that while practicing their craft baliens see trees and other parts of the landscape not as an ordinary person sees them but as houses with many people inside. One balien said that the sai are wild and do not want to go near humans but that when she sees them they are like people (that is, they look and behave like ordinary people).

Sai, of which there are an indeterminate number, may be either male or female. Each has a name corresponding to the name of a human being. They are thought to live in villages, but in a reversed world where day is night, up is down, and so on. This reversed world signifies the conscious association Taman people make between the spirit world and dream life.

The various spirits are named and categorized; they have particular characteristics and behaviors. They somewhat resemble folkloric or mythic beings, the difference being that they can actually meet and affect people. These beings are classified mainly according to their location. There are sai specific to rivers, strangling fig trees, ditches, and graveyards. Beyond that, sai may be almost anywhere. In certain cases thought of as illness, sai may appear disguised as a person to manipulate its chosen victim.[2]

In contrast to sai, there are numerous stories about antu, and encounters with them both in waking life and in dreams are reported by baliens and non-baliens alike. Thus, some implicit difference seems to be recognized between antu and sai. Unlike Taman sai, the Malay antu are said to be carried by the wind, especially after the rain. Malays, especially dukuns, have the most extensive knowledge of these spirits.

The following lists several prominent ghosts and spirits known to the Taman:

Antu Bangket (ghosts of corpses): "town ghosts." "If you are bitten, you are knocked out." "Disturbs your sleep. Can make you weak but does not cause illness or death."

Antu Gergasi: Synonymous with *Antu Kabo,* according to some informants. Other informants classified it with the "village ghosts" and said, "If you are bitten by it your bones disintegrate." Another informant said it caused kempunan.

Antu Juata: Crocodile spirit from the river, associated with *badet* caused by kempunan. Shoots objects into the person's soul. (Alternate name: *Anak Tindanum.*)

Antu Kabo: A male forest animal or ghost. "Eats your head."

Antu Karet: Sai associated with all kinds of illness, brought by a deer.

Antu Kawang: Spirit of the *kawang* (dipterocarp) tree. Sai associated with headaches.

Antu Kung: Flying lemur spirit. Passes over and makes sound of flying lemur when someone dies.

Antu Langke: Literally means "tall spirit." Sai that takes the form of an orangutan. Can cause illness or other harm. King (1976a: 135) writes that it "takes the form of a hairy giant, some 10 to 12 feet in height. It is equipped with long, sharp fangs with which it can tear and devour human flesh. It will usually attack someone who has strayed too far from the village and is lost."

Antu Saung: Associated with a kind of bird. (See King 1976a: 135–136).

Bai' Rangau: The spirit of a mythical person. Causes internal cuts in stomach or cuts off the head.

One Taman man recounted the following vivid memories of encounters he had had with ghosts.

> On one occasion, I saw a ghost in Siut [a Taman village on the Kapuas River]. It was like a man, average size. He didn't look any different from a regular person. I was bathing and I asked him what he was doing. He was also bathing, and he didn't answer. I got afraid because he just kept looking at me. After I finished bathing, I put on my clothes and was ready to go home. It was night time and there was a full moon. When I got there the ghost followed. As I walked back I kept asking him where he was going and the ghost did not answer. I went inside and told the story to my host and said maybe it was a ghost. The other man said indeed someone had died, but the *tawak* [gong] had not yet been sounded. He said, "That was a ghost you saw." Then we walked to the house [where the corpse was lying] and saw the corpse and it was wearing the same clothes as the man I had seen before.
> On another occasion I saw a ghost at Nibung [a field area upstream of Sibau Hilir]. I tied down my canoe, took off my clothes to bathe, went back, and saw a hunched man, extremely big. It was a land ghost, not a human ghost, and I went home to tell people about it. Later I went back with my friend to see it; it was still there. It looked like a person but was too big to be a real person. The moon was bright. We went to find the deputy headman to borrow a rifle to shoot it. He pulled the trigger but it didn't make a sound, even though he tried several times. This confused us and someone thought it might be a *jin* because with a ghost you can ordinarily shoot it. So he fired in the air and a bullet shot out. We tried to shoot the ghost and it didn't work. Then the headman suggested we go home. I was scared.

A few spirit beings have well-established identities. *Induayo* are ghosts of beautiful women who have hair down to their feet and pendulous breasts. They can be seen in the day if there has been rain. If there is hot rain, they come out of holes in trees. They make the sound of deer, and they lead people (especially children) astray if they have forgotten or neglected to complete an action. They are known to take people deep into the forest.

Antu Anak are ghosts that attack the heart and testicles (see Sather 1978). Some Taman consider them not to be an antu but a sai. A man who claims to have seen them described their characteristics: "Antu Anak looks like a mouse deer, about 50 centimeters high, has hair like a Westerner [*orang barat*], and long fingernails, 4 centimeters in length. Its arms are folded behind its back. It has a high-pitched voice and its call is: 'hi-hi-hi-hi.'"

Stories of Antu Anak are known throughout the Malay world, often with variant names such as *Muntianak, Matianak,* and *Pontianak.* A Malay dukun provided the following statement: "Antu Anak is Matianak (dead child). Eats blood. Makes the sound 'kak-kak-kak-kak-kak.' Itches. Causes vaginal bleeding, itchy scrotum, ceaseless bleeding if there is a cut. Eats the *cuncung* [unidentified] fruit. If you find your arms are scratched it is from Antu Anak."

Jin are considered a special category of antu and are classified as "hill ghosts." These lesser nature spirits, originally superhuman spirits or perhaps even gods to the ancient Arabians, are mentioned in the Koran and from that source entered the folk religions of those nations influenced by Islam. While jin are in nature comparable to wild beasts, they are able to appear, disappear, or change their form at will.[3] The Taman believe they are giant creatures living in the forest or hills. All jin are male, and they have only one eye, which is fire red. They are considered very dangerous, and if they attack, they can eat a person's heart. Of all the ghosts they are perhaps the most difficult to cast off. A Taman man who claimed he had often seen the jin said they live in the forest and can be seen very distinctly on the tops of trees. Some Taman informants said that Islamic dukuns have enough power that they need not fear any ghosts—except jin. A Malay dukun said that, unlike other ghosts, jin cannot be opposed, because there is no spell to neutralize them. He advised that upon meeting a jin, one should "run if possible." He added that a jin cannot hurt a person if his or her eyes are open and that an open pair of scissors prevents its entrance. However, they cannot be frightened off by the Koran, which they are able to read.

Sumangat Dualapan: The Taman Concept of Souls

Like the concepts of spirits, concepts concerning the human soul are central in understanding the balien institution. The soul is not a concern when a person is well: Then the souls are perceived as being on good behavior. It is only in dreams, illness, and death that the body and soul do not work together harmoniously (cf. Gadow 1982), and these situations may be dangerous.

The Nature and Multiple Character of Souls

The soul (*sumangat*) is not a concept of personality or of psychological structures and processes for the Taman. Rather, it is an image exactly resembling a person but capable of separating itself from the body. Baroamas Balunus (n.d.) has addressed this concept in his account of the Taman creation myth, stating that each soul goes through the same experiences and has the same face as the person to whom it belongs.

The Taman word *mintuari* refers to both the person and the body. The person is thus identified with the corporeal body in contrast with the soul, of which each person has eight (or sixteen)—*sumangat dualapan.* The uncertainty about the number of souls is the result of the ambiguity inherent in the archaic word *dualapan,* meaning "eight" but sounding like *dua lapan,* "two-eight," which implies "two times eight," or sixteen. The expression "sumangat dualapan" is always mentioned in ritualized recitations, suggesting that the words have a kind of formulaic power. Most Taman informants said that there were eight souls and that dualapan was just a rhetorical device. But some said there were indeed sixteen souls, eight good ones and eight bad or mischievous ones. One man said that people had eight good souls and eight bad ones who want them to get sick.

A middle-aged man said that according to Taman tradition there were eight souls:

> The original soul is with us always, but the others travel and can make us sick; can disturb us also. We Catholics say the souls are two: a good soul and a bad soul. The original soul lives in the back of the head, and the others exit and enter from there too. The others live in the back and get sick. If the original soul gets lost you automatically die. It's a promise from God, the person's fate.

A thirty-three-year-old man, explaining how illness is caused, said:

> Our soul travels. It meets with Antu Anak or whatever. It strikes or bites. The soul looks like ourself. When we're small there's a cavity in the crown of the head. So the soul has to leave through the fontanel also. The seven other souls are in our body. The good soul does not leave. The souls go out through the top of the head.

Other informants gave further details about the mobility of the constituent souls and their relation to illness. For example, one man stated:

> One soul never leaves, the other seven travel. They get ill and then come back. What is taken by the balien is the soul that is left behind. Only the ill souls are taken. The healthy souls are not. If the ill soul returns within a week to ten days, the person will definitely get better.

The statement of a fifty-seven-year-old man, nominally Muslim, corroborated this: "The souls that are disturbed are the wild ones. The one that stays where it belongs does not get ill."

The idea of the soul as an image of the body is understandable. But what is signified by the idea that a person has multiple souls? The principle of multiple souls means that a person can be made ill by things of which he is unconscious. The souls are not of one mind, intention, or personality: It is only the wild souls that wander off. As the psychoanalytic anthropologist Géza Róheim (1952) suggests, the naughty souls may signify the regression in the dream to an immature and unruly stage of development. By not being coordinated and united within the body, these childish souls expose one to the dangers of spirit attack and illness. The notion that the human soul is eightfold (or sixteenfold, as some maintain) seems to be a convention that does not have any deeper significance.

Dreams

Dreams are believed to be what the soul sees when it travels outside the body during sleep. They are thought to be omens about a person's fate and are often taken to signify impending illness, recovery from illness, death, or good fortune, to either the dreamer or the dreamed-of person. Dreams are the only way in which normal people (as opposed to baliens and those prone to become baliens) have contact with the spirit world. The realm of dreams is a reversal of waking life, and dreams usually mean the opposite of their manifest content.[4] Here are the interpretations of some dreams:

Illness and Fate

- If a person is ill, and someone else dreams that he or she dies, that person will get better.
- If you dream that an ill person is well dressed or has combed hair, it means that the person is "preparing to exit" (will soon die).
- If you dream of sex, it means you will get ill.[5]
- A dream of having a leech on your leg is good, meaning that an ill person will recover. But if the leech in the dream will not come off, it means that the illness will not go away and that the sick person will not recover.
- A dream that someone is laughing is bad. It means the person dreamt of will be crying. But a dream of someone crying is good.
- Dreaming that you lose a tooth is the worst dream. If it is a tooth on the left side, it means someone in your family will die; if it is on the right side, a very close family member. If it is a center tooth, it means your eldest brother or sister will die.
- If you dream about your mother, it is not good: You might get

divorced or die early. If you dream you are apart from her, it means you will always be with her in life.

- Dreams of falling trees or landslides are bad. If you have such a dream, you must cancel your plans to do something.

Fortune

- If you dream you become rich, it means you will have a financial problem.
- If you dream of eating, you will win at gambling.[6]

Animal Themes

- If you dream that you see a dog, but it doesn't bother you and you don't bother it, it means that someone wants to bother you but isn't brave enough to do anything about it. If the dog attacks you, that means you will have a fight. If in the dream you don't fight back, it means the person will take pity on you and eventually back off.
- If you dream of being bitten by a dog, punched by a person, or killed while walking, it is bad.
- If you dream that you torture an animal, it means you will have a fight.
- If you dream of talking to an animal, it is good.
- If a girl dreams she is bitten by a snake or swallowed by a crocodile, it means the relationship with the boy who wants to marry her will work out.

Bad dreams (*mui ajau*) are considered significant experiences requiring appropriate action. A daylong prohibition of travel after a bad dream is followed because of the likelihood of meeting a ghost and becoming ill.

Other bad dreams are acted upon by *mipiki*, a blessing in which a live chicken is waved behind the dreamer and his or her family members. The person reciting the blessing intones: "The bad dream is washed away by the wings of the chicken. As a chicken sweeps off the ground, so does the bad dream go away, up in the air." The dreams that have to be discharged by the mipiki ceremony are those involving conflict. An informant said that if in a dream people fight and there is no blood, the dreamer would have to undergo mipiki, but that if blood is shed in the dream, a legal proceeding would be enacted. Another typical dream that must be sent away by mipiki is one of being in a boat that capsizes.

By contrast, a dream in which the dreamer travels to a field, gets lost, or cannot return implies another kind of danger and must be treated by a balien. Dreams in which dead people are seen require balien seances to locate and retrieve the soul of the dreamer.

Implicit in the Taman notion of dreaming as soul travel is the idea that dreams are potentially dangerous: The souls leaving the body meet spirit beings that may cause harm. Infants, who have a high mortality rate, are thought to be at the greatest risk. Consequently, Taman attach charms to the hammocks in which they sleep. Sexual dreams are also considered potentially dangerous, as they connote intimacy with spirits. Such dreams, if brought to light, could result in treatment by a balien and ultimately initiation into the balien group (see Chapter 5).

Death (and Near Death)

The notion of death as "a promise from God" is generalized, and this maxim is often mentioned in speeches at funerals, meaning that death is fated. Death is conceived of as a journey rather than an instantaneous event (cf. Harrisson 1962; Metcalf 1982). Contact with the body of a dead person is not considered singularly polluting; however, the interference of the dead with the affairs of the living is considered dangerous.

In the following account a man interpreted a dream of his dead daughter as an encounter with her ghost.

> When my daughter died I was very sad. She had not been sick. I still remember her fondly. When she was buried I dreamed that I walked very far until I was covered with sweat. Then I saw her dressed in beautiful clothes. There were four policemen there. They asked me where I was going and called me "sir" (*Pak*). I said I wanted to see my daughter. They asked me where I had seen her. I said I saw her talking happily with many people. Then they said, "Please enter," and I entered the house. I saw the girl sitting in the center, as if in a government ceremony. Then a policeman guarding the door asked me where I was going. He let me in. I asked a person behind her, who said, "You cannot come in here." "Why not?" I asked. He answered, "The problem is, your daughter has already gone to heaven, led by God. Please go home, don't stay here." "How can I go? I just want to talk to her a minute." "You can't," the person said. "Then if I can't, where should I sit?" I asked. Then I woke up.

The informant considered this a good dream, because he was told that his daughter had already gone to heaven and that he should go back home to normal earthly life.

The Taman say that at death the soul travels to Bukit Tilung, a mountain in Mandai Subdistrict. There is believed to be a beautiful house there, in which the souls of all dead people live happily, dressed in fine clothes. Yang Suka presides and determines who can enter the house.[7]

There are some reports of dead people returning from the land of the dead (perhaps by chance, all the reports concern women). These stories recount the journey to the land of the dead and the judgment by Yang Suka, and they epitomize the notion that the dead prosper in finer, more luxurious circumstances than obtain in earthly life. These stories are important because they show how near-death experiences of the Taman are configured within their eschatology, adding to our understanding of the role of culture and belief systems in structuring such mystical experiences. Tom Harrisson (1965: 288–290) provides a remarkable account of "the girl who died twice." In the story the girl (from Lunsa village on the Kapuas River) encounters sixteen friendly people (eight men and eight women), who take her along a great road.[8] They come across several obstacles until finally they arrive at the great longhouse on Bukit Tilung, where the girl is greeted with ceremony. She meets her deceased relatives, who are unfriendly to her. She then meets Yang Suka, who appears as a handsome but otherwise ordinary man. According to the girl, "If we come from a good family and are without sins he kindly takes care of us. But if we have committed sins during our lifetime, we are punished, directly, in front of many people. When this person came near me he said: 'The time has not yet come for you to come here and you will be coming later'" (Harrisson 1965: 290). At that point the girl felt as if she were falling from the longhouse and she awoke, much to the amazement of the mourners at her funeral.

I collected similar stories from two people in Sibau Hilir. One young man told me the story of Grandmother Sano, which is very similar to but less detailed than the incident described by Harrisson.

> A woman was dead for two nights and a day. Then she woke up, was weak for a while, asked for food, and told her story. She said there was a wide, beautiful, clean road that she walked on. Many people followed her: young and old, male and female, people she knew and people she did not know. After about 3 kilometers there was a fork in the road. Many people took the road to the right. Someone informed her that that road was for people who had sinned, and that she should take the left-hand road. After half a kilometer there was a big log that became the street. People in front of her were happy to go on this log, and they had no trouble jumping up on it. But she could not, and kept falling. Then she woke up and was already in the coffin. In those days Sibau was still animist. She lived for twenty years after that event. She died for real six years ago.

Another informant told the following story:

> My older sister died, and an hour later came back to life. She said the land of the dead was more *ramai* [in this context, "friendly" or "happy"] than here, they had enough clothes. She didn't want to come back but there was someone there who told her to go back. She said the people in heaven wear white from head to toe. The person who told her to go home was a man, but she did not know his identity.

Illness

Illness is conceived of primarily as an injury to one or more of the multiple and separable souls. Since the soul is not a psychological concept affiliated specifically with personality or consciousness, this concept of illness does not imply that illness is in the mind; nor does it refer to mental illness or psychological distress. Spirits may attack the soul by shooting an object at it, mutilating (e.g., biting or stabbing) it, or decapitating it. Spirit attack may result in simple illness or fever (*bangkar*) or in illness or pain (both called *pais*) specific to a certain body part. These illnesses are treated by the balien with *bubut,* a simple and common therapy in which stones are stroked over the body to extract the disease, represented materially by tiny pebbles or other objects "plucked" out of the body that drop into a bowl held against the patient.

In the case of more advanced illnesses, the balien first performs bubut, then seeks to determine the location of the soul. This procedure suggests that the soul has been separated from the body, is missing, and may have been seized by a spirit. For the wild soul to wander from the body is not in itself considered pathological, but if it has not returned within a few days, it may be lost. The further the soul has traveled, the more difficult it is to return, and if it wanders as far as Bukit Tilung, the person could die. In cases of serious illness caused by spirit attack, it is thought that the soul has been captured and is being tormented in revenge for harm done to that spirit.

Another way spirits may cause illness is to disturb the soul. These disturbances, or afflictions, may be tests by spirits. They are thought to connote deliberate torment and victimization but also, paradoxically, love. While spirit attack is motivated by revenge, spirit affliction has no rationale in terms of the victim's behavior. Instead, it is attributed to the irrational fancies or passions of the spirit or spirits. Even though illnesses of spirit affliction have no motive, they may well have a purpose, in the sense that the victims may be considered selected for initiation as a balien. (This process is discussed in detail in Chapter 5.)

The balien's techniques for curing illness suggest three categories of illness, arranged in order of increasing seriousness. Although there are seven balien ceremonies (including *menyarung,* the initiation ceremony), they amount to three basic procedures: (1) removal of a spirit being or projectile object sent by a spirit; (2) recall and restoration of an errant soul; and (3) neutralization of free spirits that disturb a person. The implicit causes underlying these therapies are (1) projectile assault on the soul, (2) loss or capture of the soul, and (3) disturbance of the soul (see Table 4.1).

These treatments are not fully correlated to the concepts of illness causation. In particular, soul loss or soul capture is not considered to be the cause of illness or even the means by which a spirit causes illness. Rather, as I suggest in Table 4.1 (see also Bernstein n.d.) soul loss or soul capture is simply an attribute of advanced cases of illness by spirit attack that must be treated. Moreover, spirit attack is not always conceptualized as a projectile attack. Balien therapies do not necessarily treat the underlying cause; rather, they treat certain attributes related to how illness was incurred. For example,

Table 4.1 **The Progression of Balien Ceremonies in Relation to Concepts of Illness**

Illness category	Underlying cause	Treatment (Balien ceremony)	Attribute treated
Pais layu-layu or *dawawa jalu*	Balien destiny	*Menyarung*	Balien destiny
Pais layu-layu or *dawawa jalu*	Spirit disturbance	*Mengadengi*	Spirit disturbance
Pais layu-layu	Spirit attack and/or spirit disturbance	*Menindoani* or *tabak buse*	Soul capture
Badi or *kempunan*	Spirit attack	*Malai*	Soul capture
Badi or *kempunan*	Spirit attack	*Mangait*	Soul loss
Luka sai/ Bangkar	Spirit attack	*Bubut*	Projectile attack

a patient may be treated by object extraction even if the illness is thought to have been caused by frontal assault. The range of therapies also suggests that levels of increasingly advanced therapies correlate to increasingly severe illness. However, illnesses caused by spirit attack are classified in terms of their underlying causes rather than their immediate manifestations. In the case of "simple" illnesses treated by object extraction, the particular details of the treatment may label the illness, as described in Chapter 6. "Soul loss," however, does not identify any kind of serious illness or its causes.

The relationship between spirit attack and spirit disturbance is ambiguous. In general, illnesses of spirit disturbance are those previously treated as illnesses of spirit attack (and perhaps another cause before that) that have been reinterpreted in light of either a significant pattern of reoccurrence or a relevant dream or daydream (usually erotic). In other cases the victim, though not suffering from any other condition of illness, may continually meet and be confused or disturbed by an apparition. These kinds of illness are treated by ceremonies in which spirits are neutralized, called mengadengi. While this notion of illness resulting from spirit disturbance is very different from the ideas of object intrusion and soul loss, the procedures of object removal and seance to locate the soul are incorporated into the mengadengi ceremony. This suggests that the increasing levels of illness are cumulative. Thus, an illness of spirit disturbance has the attributes of projectile attack, soul loss, soul capture, and victimization.

In biomedical terms, illnesses of spirit disturbance are not more serious than illnesses of spirit attack. Indeed, acute illnesses would be treated as spirit attack rather than spirit disturbance. But spirit disturbance is the more serious category in terms of the perceived threat to the patient's soul.

Illness and death are not always attributed to spirit attack, and interpretations of the cause of illness may be revised. That is, one may go to a clinic or consult a dukun before or after balien treatment. Also, it is recognized that illness may be the result of several factors at once.

Illnesses Attributed to Spirit Attack

Internal Cuts (Luka Ilalam, Luka Sai)

Disease may enter a person in several ways: by projectile attack, in which a spirit with a blowdart inflicts a cut; by a spirit entering the body; or by direct attack, in which a spirit punches, spears, stabs, claws, or bites. In all cases, it is one of the multiple and separable souls, not the physical body, that has been attacked by the spirit, but the attack causes the body to ache. An informant said that the spirit Grandfather Rangau attacks victims by cutting their heads off, but "the head is not severed and there is no wound, because it is the soul that is attacked." The assault is not felt at the moment it happens, but afterward sharp pain may be felt briefly.

For the most part, explanations of "internal cut" or "being stabbed by a spirit" are applied to simple illnesses (bangkar) or body part illnesses (e.g., stomachache, toothache, or backache). However, one illness often associated with "internal cuts" or "attack by a demon," called najam in Malay or badet in Taman, is more complex. This is a cramplike pain in the abdomen or chest that may travel to different parts of the torso (this movement is considered significant); shortness of breath is also symptomatic.

If simple treatments have proven ineffective, or if there are complicating signs (from dreams for example), illness from a spirit is explained in terms of the spirit's motivation to cause harm. While internal cuts may be present, a balien may detect a more serious illness, either badi or kempunan, which is associated with soul loss and is attributed to a motivated attack.

Badi *or* dabalas jalu

Among the Taman and the Upper Kapuas Malay, badi refers specifically to the revenge by a ghost, goblin, or other spirit for causing it harm. That the act was unintentional or unconscious is of no concern to the spirit. In fact, the victim of badi need not have personally inflicted the pain to be susceptible to a spirit attack; he or she might simply have the same name as the spirit being. The Taman expression *pambalasan jalu,* "revenge of a demon (or spirit being)," has the same meaning as the Malay *sakit badi,* "badi illness." This concept of badi must be differentiated from the notion that is prevalent in the Malay peninsula of badi as an "evil principle which may have entered a man who unguardcdly touchcd a dcad animal or bird from which the badi has not yet been expelled" (Skeat 1900: 427).[9]

Badi as an etiological category has on the surface diverse varieties and causes, underlying different kinds of acute illness. The main types of badi are from fire—specifically from hearths built outside or in temporary shelters (*badi api*)—a stake in the ground (*badi pancak, badi turos*), ants (*badi semadak, badi lumantik*), cats (*badi pusa'*), and corpses (*badi bangkai*). Fire badi and stake badi are caused by spirits living underground that have been injured through fire or stakes.

The classification of badi illness is based on the way the symptoms correlate to the way it might have been caused. Fire badi is an inflammation; this malady may be contracted when a person sets a fire at a campsite or rice field. Black-ant badi burns and itches; it is considered by some informants to be a category of fire badi caused when a person burns a fire in an ants' nest in rotten wood. Stake badi is sharp internal pain and digestive difficulties, a stabbing pain in revenge for the spirit being stabbed with a stake in the ground. It might be caused not only by planting a stake but by removing or burning one. Cat badi may take the form of weakness and dizziness. But as one informant said, "If we kill a cat, its soul takes revenge. Depending on how it died, that's how we will be made to suffer. All animals in the ground can take revenge."

The following is a case in which a young woman's death was attributed to badi:

> A young woman who died after having a miscarriage is said later to be the victim of dabalas jalu. She was in a camp with her husband while she was pregnant, and a snake was found under the house, that he killed. My informant says all kinds of animals—snakes and monkeys, for example—can take revenge in this way. The animal doesn't care who killed it. The point is, it has the same name.

Prototypical symptoms of badi are infection (boils or abscesses) and shortness of breath. However, any malady, regardless of the specific symptoms, could be from badi. Miscarriages, measles, malaria, rheumatism, cancer, and digestive, urinary, or genital troubles are among the illnesses caused by badi. Congenital deformity is explained as badi having set in during gestation. Even those diseases that most informants said were not from badi, such as herpes (*antumelet*), were thought by a few people to be possibly from badi if a balien or dukun could cure it. Here is what one man in his forties said about this matter:

> When the *manang* [the Iban term for balien] does the *mangait* [ceremony to locate and call back the soul], she knows whether measles is real measles or badi. Many things can be badi, but dysentery isn't. The proof is

in the balien's diagnosis. The balien is the only one [who knows]. Cancer may be from badi, or may be from punti. If cancer grows from a boil it may be called badi. If a wart becomes cancer, it is not badi. Fungal itch is not badi. If it becomes ringworm, it's still not badi. Herpes is badi. It can be medicated [treated by bubut] by a balien; it can be cured.

This man shared the opinion of most informants that the majority of skin diseases could not be from badi, but if they become infections (boils), badi may be suspected. But he was in the minority in saying herpes or cancer could be from badi. Most informants attributed cancerous tumors to growths from within the body. Since these are internal causes, they are incompatible with balien treatment.

Not all infections or illnesses can be attributed to badi. Yohanes cut his leg on some wood, and the wound became infected some days later. After he realized he could no longer ignore the condition, he treated himself with common herbal remedies, to draw out pus. He changed the salves five times a day, and he also used some sangka' he had inherited from his father, one of which was a medicine for infections. He wanted to go to a doctor in town but could not afford to do so. Since the infection did not clear up promptly, he decided to put medicine on it, possibly with the persuasion of others. Even though Yohanes said that badi could cause a similar infection, he did not consider bringing his problem to a balien or seeking another magical cure. As he put it, "This is a cut. The balien cures disease." Since the ultimate cause of the ailment was a known action Yohanes himself had committed, it was impossible for him to attribute the resulting illness to an unseen cause.

Kempunan

Kempunan (also called *kaponan*) refers to danger created by failing to complete an intended action or carry out an expected one. It is closely linked to the concept of badi: Kempunan can cause the same kinds of illnesses, and both are treated by a balien using the same means. Like badi, kempunan is an illness caused by spirit attack. Belief in kempunan is more widespread (or at least more widely documented) than belief in badi (Bernstein 1994, n.d.).

Kempunan is an integral part of everyday culture in the entire Upper Kapuas region, not only in Taman villages, and is related to ingrained norms of behavior and etiquette. I learned about kempunan early in my research among the Taman. Before I moved to a Taman village, a Dutch priest long stationed in the Embaloh area of Benua Martinus explained to me the delicate art of rejecting food or drink. The way to decline an offer of food, he said, was to touch it lightly with the fingertips and then touch one's own chest or lips. Doing this is the same as accepting the food, and it defuses any feeling of offense. While performing this action (called *melepos*) the Taman say "Pos, pos."[10] Accepting food (or drink, tobacco, or betel quid) in this way is considered not a rejection but a completion of an action or plan.

I found that among the Taman, when food or drink was being consumed, it was offered to everyone in the vicinity. At weddings, girls would approach each male celebrant sitting in a row and place a bit of food in his mouth. At other ceremonies, a man would pass each participant a cup he would fill with liquor that the person was expected to imbibe. Refusal under these circumstances would be awkward. I once noticed a spoonful of rice being passed around a longhouse veranda as people touched the spoon and then their lips. On another occasion, a man berated me for eating a plate of food without offering it to the people in the room, as if I were worried that the people would eat up my food. The implication was that I was exposing the others to kempunan. An informant once let me in on a secret about etiquette: "If my wife is inside cooking and I am in front with my friends she may not call me in to eat unless all the other people are invited too. Otherwise, if there is not enough food, she will eat alone." This custom is explained by concern about exposure to kempunan.

Kempunan is essentially a situation of danger created when a person has a desire for something but neglects to satisfy it. This neglect is viewed as failure to complete an action. There are several kinds of kempunan, corresponding to a range of frustrated urges, the most prototypical being that for a specific food or drink. For example, a twenty-seven-year-old man told me about his experience with kempunan, which began when he neglected to satisfy a desire he had to eat fried rice.

> Three years ago my left leg was swollen in a flexed position and could not move. Because of that I could not walk. This happened because I forgot to eat fried rice. I just woke up one day and found I could not walk. My behavior the previous day caused the illness. I went to two dukuns who both tried to cure me by rubbing sangka' (antidotes) on the bad leg, but it did not help. Then I went to a doctor in Putussibau who gave me an injection of vitamin B complex. Then I went to yet another man who tried to cure me with oils like the previous two. Finally I tried another Malay dukun who treated the leg by rubbing it with a rhinoceros tooth and a stone dipped in water, while reciting verses from the Koran. Little by little the leg got better. Finally in nine months it was better, but not a hundred percent better. I still want to find another healer to cure me.

Failure to carry out the intention to bathe can also induce a kempunan attack. The urge to bathe is not specific—unlike the desire for a specific food or drink—but bathing is a liminal activity, and as with eating and drinking, a person who is bathing may be thoroughly absorbed. Sexual desire is sometimes mentioned in connection with kempunan. Like the desire for food or drink, it very likely has a specific object. Some informants said that if one's mind is occupied in this way by a certain person, it will definitely lead to kempunan unless a sexual relationship is achieved.

Kempunan attacks may be precipitated by another kind of omission. If a person is not offered or invited to share some commodity being consumed by another—be it food, drink, tobacco, or betel nut—that person is exposed to kempunan by not being able to accept it. In offering whatever is being consumed to all people on the premises, a person intends to protect them from the dangers of kempunan. In both cases—neglecting to satisfy one's own urge and neglecting to partake of food or drink being enjoyed by another person—kempunan is believed to follow from failure to complete an action. Unlike badi, which is caused without any intention, kempunan relates to deliberate activity, and thus it can be prevented by observing prescriptive norms. Kempunan-related danger and attacks occur when rules for behavior are not observed. Thus, kempunan is caused by the violation of a taboo.

Kempunan is a form of spirit attack much like badi, except that the revenge generally takes the form of an accident rather than an illness. Bites by snakes and other venomous (*berbisa*) animals, such as centipedes and scorpions, and by other animals like bears and crocodiles—all real dangers—are considered the most characteristic result of kempunan. In fact, the Taman believe there is no plausible explanation for animal bites other than kempunan.

Animals are explicitly associated by the Taman with invisible animal spirits. The stinging attacks of animals such as snakes, centipedes, and scorpions are considered analogous to the attack of a spirit. By the logic of kempunan as spirit attack, if illness rather than an animal bite occurs after a person has been exposed to kempunan, then an animal spirit bit the person, causing the illness. Such an illness may be cured by a balien. But illness or bodily trauma following the attack of a living animal, though caused by kempunan, cannot be treated by a balien.[11]

Kempunan is only incidentally related to beliefs and values about health and illness; it is part of an all-encompassing set of attitudes about harmony and the ordering of things or actions—the notion of a proper or right way of doing things. Kempunan orders and in a way ritualizes private behavior. Only behavior carried out according to culturally appropriate norms of completeness are fully constituted as actions.

The person who neglects to receive food may not have consciously experienced any craving for it. Acceptance of food is part of a norm of sociability; failure to accept, whether accidental or not, could cause harm to the other party. Therefore, kempunan is more puzzling as an explanation of illness than is badi. Unlike badi, which follows some action, kempunan is set in motion when a person neglects to carry out an action. Such actions appear to have nothing to do with spirits. If kempunan is a category of spirit attack, the problem is to determine why a spirit would be motivated to attack a person who has acted in such a manner. Does such behavior offend it morally, or is it impelled to take revenge for having been harmed directly, as in badi?

The kinds of actions that result in badi and kempunan seem unrelated. Badi is caused by an action that has caused harm to a spirit, even though it was not intended to do so. The liable person may have been either aware or unaware of committing the action; thus, a distinction may be made between unintended and unwitting action. Kempunan, however, may be caused by a desired, intended, or contemplated action that is not carried out. But such a circumstance is not the only cause; failure to receive or accept, whatever the internal state of intention or desire, can also result in kempunan. The danger of denial extends beyond an individual's intention or awareness at the level of ego, to a larger set of participants. That set is not only social but cosmic, since it includes spirits.

To understand kempunan, and particularly the "locus of responsibility" in cases attributed to it (Foster 1976), it is necessary to accept the notion that "action" begins before there is physical movement, possibly with a scenario in the mind or a pre-existing situation to which one must respond in a certain way. In these terms, human action is not necessarily a physical movement, but it is consequential. An action is something for which a person is responsible and may be held accountable. The actions that must be completed in the appropriate ways are those that relate to bodily gratification and frustration. Failure to complete them (consciously, unintentionally, or unwittingly) exposes a person to kempunan, a vulnerability to revenge attack by a spirit. The main concern in kempunan beliefs seems to be orality.[12] This may be the prototype of the kempunan concept, since the attack made in revenge (by either a spirit or a living animal) is prototypically a bite.

Physical manifestations of illness alone are not diagnostic of whether illness is the result of badi or kempunan. The attribution of illness to spirit attack is related to a larger set of variables involving relations with family members and other associates as well as past activities. However, there may be a viable alternative explanation to spirit attack, including external and internal causes, in any individual case of illness. We shall consider first the external sources resulting in illness that cannot be treated by the balien.

The Wind as a Source of Illness

In Malay belief, wind (*angin*—the Taman word is *soangin*) is said to be controlled by devils (*setan*) and to carry with it many dangerous ghosts.[13] Some believe that wind is indistinguishable from the ghosts it carries. Besides containing dangerous spirits, the wind can enter the body—for example, while the person is bathing or walking—causing illness. In the hierarchy of winds, *angin ahmal* is the strongest and most dangerous. Wind from ghosts is said to originate from the hills. A Malay healer, citing "scripture," stated that "Reban mountain is where you [wind] live, Majapahit land is where you originated." Wind can enter the body through the hands, feet, jaws, or wherever there is pain. Several techniques for ridding the body of wind are described in Chapter 3. Gastritis caused by wind is called *dugal* by Malay dukuns, who scorn the balien's bubut treatment for such illness. The dukuns believe that abdominal pain is not caused by spirits but is instead the result of the blood not flowing because hot wind has entered the body. The dukuns disagree about whether hot and cold winds have different effects. One dukun firmly believed that ghosts were brought by the hot wind after a rain, while another disagreed. The Malay dukuns do attribute sudden weakness to wind. In the words of one, "If you come home from fishing and are hit by the wind, you cannot walk."

Many ordinary illnesses like headaches, stomachaches, and rheumatism are attributed to wind. Rheumatism was explained as originating from water being hit by wind; bathing with such water may result in illness. Some Taman people think that such illnesses are best treated by patent medicines obtained from pharmacies.

The wind can also be a vehicle for people to send illness, in the form of intoned spells (*pulung*). As one informant said, "Pulung can fly." People knowledgeable about Malay medicine called these spells "false wind" or "man-made wind" and said they were far more dangerous than natural wind. Pulung was compared to voodoo. For the Taman, pulung is the exception to the rule that any illness is treatable by the balien or other traditional medicine: Illness "from antu anak can be bubut-ed; what can't be bubut-ed is pulung. Pulung is automatic, there are momentary shivers; one can die; cannot speak. It cannot be cured by injection." The only effective treatment for pulung is the appropriate counterspell or antidote.

Illnesses Attributed to Internal Causes

Internally caused diseases are not necessarily minor; however, they cannot be explained as resulting from an external cause, which is the standard etiology of disease. Many skin diseases, coughs, fevers, and mental illnesses are thought to come from within the body. Typical explanations of these ailments include dirty blood, drinking unclean water, heredity, contagion, epidemics, eating hot or cold food, or "snapped nerves" (*putus urat saraf*).

Dirty blood seems to be a residual category for infectious states that the Taman and Malay do not understand. One Taman man said it refers to a woman's menstrual blood. Another said that the sign of dirty blood is frequent headaches. One informant said that very painful infections called *isi-uranan* (meaning "snakebite" because of the severity of the pain) were the result of dirty blood: "Dirty blood can be cured by a balien, depending on the desire of the person, if it is fitting."

Skin diseases are regarded as both contagious and hereditary. Epidemics are labeled "seasonal" diseases, and are said categorically not to be from badi. Certain rashes are known to result from contact with irritating substances, like the sap of some kinds of trees or the secretions of a sort of ant. Some informants said that certain skin diseases could be caused by eating foods classified as "hot." I never heard of any actual instances of disease being attributed to hot or cold food, however, when curing sick people, healers would mention certain foods prohibited on these grounds. Other food prohibitions derive from ancestral injunctions. The idea of illness resulting from the consumption of dirty water or contact with it is widely accepted: stomachaches (especially diarrhea) and coughs are attributed to this.

The Malay dukun Rachman said tuberculosis was hereditary. Considering the matter further, he commented that it was caused not by poisoning but "because people are not clean, what they eat is not clean."[14]

Illnesses considered constitutional (for example, high blood pressure) are thought treatable only by doctors' medicine. Informants who had been diagnosed as having high blood pressure or who believed they suffered from it sought relief from traditional medicine, but the illness kept recurring.[15] This experience may have made them weary (and wary) of traditional (non-biomedical) forms of medicine.

An interesting category in disease etiology is malaria. The early symptoms of malaria—alternating shivers and fevers—are known as *dajulung,* which can develop into a more serious illness, *mangura.* Some informants thought that only young men, and not the whole population, were prone to contract mangura. The word "malaria" is used to explain the cause of certain "conditional" illnesses that are not congenital but begin at a certain time. Many cases of mental abnormality are explained as originating in malaria; others are said to originate in transgressing a prohibition, such as the prohibitions of treatment imposed by a healer.

The following explanation was given for the fact that a sixteen-year-old boy was still in sixth grade and apparently mentally slow.

> Before he took the test to graduate from elementary school he sought mystical knowledge [probably a spell or mantra] to help him graduate. He went to a dukun to get medicine to make him intelligent. But he went crazy. Then he was treated in the mengadengi (stone-catching) ceremony by eight baliens to make him normal again. When he was crazy he ran around, said he heard voices, and ran into the forest.
> The dukun gave him the medicine correctly, but the boy ignored the prohibition. The main prohibition was pork. [Apparently connoting general Muslim prohibition of pork.] Also, he was not allowed to walk under the house or cross a clothesline. Because the boy disregarded the proscriptions, he's in sixth grade again. Previously he was of average intelligence.

A number of informants told me that madness (*baungau*) could be from "snapped nerves" (putus urat saraf). The dukun Rachman was the only one able to elaborate as to what that illness means: "The blood in the head is dirty, so the nerve breaks. The blood is not red but black. It can cause madness. The nerves cannot work because of the dirty blood. This is treated by cupping." Yet another nervous or behavioral disorder, epilepsy, is thought to be internally caused. Conceptually, it is part of a cluster of illnesses including *karawan* (swollen glands in the neck and cheeks, possibly mumps) and *ketiap* (swelling or a tumor in the groin). Both of these illnesses are believed to be the result of *sekitam,* which is probably a contraction of the Malay *sakit hitam,* literally "black disease." The first symptom of sekitam is that the arms turn black and become itchy. But *sekitam* and the Taman equivalent, *karangan,* soon develop into a pattern of sudden illness, dizziness, and fainting. The greatest danger, according to informants, is that a person bathing alone is prone to faint in the water and drown.

If not treated, karawan leads to karawan bawi ("pig karawan"); the Malay term *gila babi* ("pig madness") is also used. Linda Kimball mentions pig madness in her study of Malay medicine in Brunei (the reader may note a similarity not only to epilepsy but to rabies):

> "Pig madness" differs from other insanities. It is not a bad illness because the patient does not hurt others although he often kills himself. Pig madness gets its name from the fact that the victim falls down, lies rigidly, roots around the floor like a pig, trembles, foams at the mouth, and sometimes swallows his tongue. The patient is unconscious. . . . Attacks come on suddenly, sometimes in the midst of eating or swimming. When the attack comes the victim looks for water, jumping in if he finds it. He may swim if he knows how but swims aimlessly rather than toward the shore, hence the mortality from drowning. (Kimball 1979: 270)

This cluster of illnesses is said by the Taman to be curable only by Malay dukuns. However, the prognosis of karawan is very unfavorable, and it is thought likely that the victim will suffer a lingering death.

The Explanation of Illness

In explaining illness the Taman may refer to one of several etiologies, but an essential distinction is drawn between illness originating within the body and illness originating externally. Illnesses that can be attributed to a discernable external cause and those thought to come from within the body are considered to be within the purview of government medicine, including store-bought medicine. However, if the cause of illness is unknown (as is usually the case), or if illness appears in some way to be out of the ordinary—either occurring suddenly or coming and going inexplicably—relief may be sought in a variety of folk therapies. It is here that the concepts of badi and kempunan, which embody folk ideas of illness and harm, come into play. If illness does not fit into a frame of expectation of being from an identifiable cause—eating spoiled food or stepping on a thorn—then an external cause seems plausible. The expectations of the sufferer, and perhaps even more of his or her family members, account for the attribution of illness to spirits, human action (poisons or spells), wind, or another factor.

The etiological concepts are legitimized in different ways in the various medical complexes to which Taman have access. The selection of a particular mode of illness causation entails a relationship with a certain kind of healer, be it a Taman balien, a Malay dukun, a doctor or nurse, a peripatetic herbalist, or the owner of a charm or magical antidote. Over a period of time, illness may be interpreted and treated in a number of different ways based on a number of different etiological premises. Not only Taman baliens but several Malay dukuns partake in a belief system wherein badi or kempunan may cause illness; both kinds of healers may diagnose and treat those illnesses, though they use different techniques because the underlying rationales of their therapeutic systems are divergent. Each kind of healing invokes a different set of meanings that shapes the course of treatment and interpretation of illness, making it social by creating "sickness episodes" (Frankenberg 1980; Young 1976a). The process of attributing a specific cause—external or internal—to a case of illness situates that case in a context of socially recognizable meanings and delimits the range of appropriate treatment strategies and possible outcomes.

Notes

1. "Illness" has been defined by Eisenberg (1977: 11) as "a person's perceptions and experiences of socially disvalued states including, but not limited to, disease." "Disease," in turn, "refers to abnormalities in the structure and/or function of organs and organ systems; pathological states whether or not they are culturally recognized; the area of the biomedical model" (Eisenberg 1977: 9).

2. Pais layu-layu and dawawa jalu, described in Chapter 5.

3. For further information on jin in Islam see Gimlette 1971: 26-36; Macdonald and Massé 1965.

4. The careful reader will notice that a few dreams are interpreted as having meanings parallel to their manifest content. The only explanation I can think of is that other interpretations may be too unpalatable to contemplate.

5. A reference to spirit disturbance and affliction. See Chapter 5.

6. This dream was collected early in 1986, but the introduction of a soccer sweepstakes (*Porkas*) and another lottery (*Dana*) to the area in 1987 sharpened people's consciousness of the possible meaning of dreams. People would bet on number or letter combinations that came to them in dreams.

7. Harrisson (1965: 342, n. 104) likens him to Saint Peter, though the Taman in general claimed that Yang Suka means God.

8. Compare the translation of sumangat dualapan as "two times eight souls."

9. Endicott (1970: 66) quotes several similar definitions of badi, none of which is pertinent to the concept of badi in Taman or Upper Kapuas Malay ethnomedicine, except for one mentioned in R. J. Wilkinson's *Malay-English*

Dictionary (1901: 78): "the infection of a disease." Skeat describes a practice based on a premise approaching the Taman concept of badi (specifically, badi api): "The hearth-fire (*api dapor*) must never be stepped over (*di-langkah-nya*) nor must the rice-pot which stands upon it, as in the latter case the person who does so will be 'cursed by the Rice'" (Skeat 1900: 319). Also similar is this practice cited in Hose and McDougall's *Pagan Tribes of Borneo*: "Among the Iban, if a man finds that someone has deposited dirt about his premises he takes a few burning sticks and thrusting them into the dirt, says: 'Now let them suffer the pains of dysentery'" (Hose and McDougall 1912, II: 40, 118; cited in Róheim 1930:12).

10. Possibly derived from the Malay *melepas,* meaning "release," a basic ritual procedure.

11. A person bitten or stung by an animal is considered to be in a state of ritual danger, as evidenced by the prohibition of such a person being brought indoors before full recovery. Transgressing this prohibition is believed to be fatal for the victim.

12. The theme of orality returns in the reinterpretation of illness as spirit disturbance, described in Chapter 5.

13. This concept of wind is different from that of the Terengganu Malays described by Laderman (1991), for whom wind is an internal phenomenon.

14. Probably a reference to the fact that the non-Muslim Dayaks do not observe Islamic dietary laws.

15. The Taman do not know how to measure blood pressure, but the notion of high blood pressure (*darah tinggi*) is widespread, and many people presume that they have this condition.

5

Becoming a Balien

The origin of the balien is the power of spirits (*dewa*). The signs of someone becoming a balien are: lust for the devil (*setan iblis*), dreams of being
taken by the devil, no appetite for food, and an unsettled mind.
—Conversation with two Taman men

A person does not become a balien by receiving training but through
induction in an initiation ceremony. To understand the nature of balienism
as a medical discipline, it is necessary to grasp the fact that people become
baliens through an involuntary process, unlike the practitioners of pharmaceutical cures, who acquire medical knowledge for purposes of gain. While
uncommon or oil-based medicines used by ordinary people are mystified by
being kept secret, baliens are people of known status, initiated in public ceremonies. Unlike the secretive nonprofessionalized medicinal curers in their
society, they are obliged to cure when called upon.

The predisposing condition leading to a person's inauguration as a
balien is inferred from dreams and physical and behavioral signs (including
some commonly recognized as illness) that suggest an ineluctable destiny to
join this healing vocation.

Predisposing Conditions and the Reinterpretation of Illness

People become baliens because of a condition interpreted as an illness. Most
commonly, baliens experienced sexually arousing dreams or fantasies
before initiation. In these dreams, a person may find him- or herself being
pursued by an aggressive suitor or lover. The person then experiences a
longing for the fantasy figure and may see apparitions of it in waking life. If
recurring, such dreams and fantasies are not considered to be caused by the
subject's own desires or imagination. Instead, they result from the person's
having been "targeted" as a victim by a spirit who is in love with the person.
The person may therefore deny any active role in making up the fantasy.

The object appearing in the dream or fantasy may resemble one's own spouse or another known person of the opposite sex. Informants describe the emotion as love—a compulsive emotional attachment to the object. The subject feels an uncontrollable desire for the image even when it is eventually realized that it is an apparition and not an actual person. In fact, the actual person whom the apparition resembles may not elicit the same response, and people suffering from this disorder maintain that the figure in their vision is more handsome or more beautiful than the real-life person.

An ordinary illness, such as stomach cramps, may be reinterpreted in light of a dream or fantasy as a disturbance by a spirit, particularly if it recurs in a pattern corresponding to the dreams. Most baliens said that their illnesses prior to initiation were mild or ordinary and were not alarming in themselves.

The narrative of a man who had been treated days earlier by baliens in a ceremony (mengadengi) to catch disturbing spirits exemplifies clearly the dissociation of one's own will from fantasy that is characteristic of this illness.

> Before my illness I frequently dreamed of a certain girl. When I saw the living person, I did not have any feeling toward her. This was because I was falling in love with a spirit rather than an actual person. This is typical of someone who is destined to become a balien. She could touch me but I could not touch her. I would see the apparition and want to follow it instead of my wife. The first time I was sick I was in my rice field planting something, walking about 10 meters ahead of my wife. Then I saw the girl who had been in my dreams. She wrapped her arms around me, but when I tried to return the embrace she was gone and I saw her somewhere else. I followed her and tried to catch up with her, but she disappeared again only to reappear somewhere else. My wife pointed this [his odd behavior] out and asked, "Where are you going?" Only then did I realize that I had been distracted from my work, and I returned to my wife. After this I longed for the girl. That night she came again. According to other people I began dancing, but I was not aware of this myself.[1]

The experience is one of seduction, but it may be frightening. The person may feel conflict about the fantasy, as in one case in which a woman, Bolom, later initiated as a balien, reported that at first she was frightened by a dream in which an unknown man asked her to make love to him and threatened her with a knife when she refused. Subsequently, however, she fell in love with this man and began to refuse her husband sexually out of preference for the dreamed figure.

These dreams and apparitions are thought to lead to insanity if not treated appropriately by shamans who catch the intruding spirit. One informant mentioned that a possible expression of such madness is to run wild in the forest. I was told about such a case by a man whose kinsman disappeared for two weeks, lost in the forest. When he returned he said he had been taken away by three beautiful women (spirits): One grabbed him while the others held him down.

Besides the erotic dream or fantasy, other symptoms of spirit affliction are dreams, anxieties, or delusions concerning food, often coinciding with eating disorders and noticeable weight loss. For example, Bolom had dreamed that she alone, in a group of people, had been offered raw food, while the others were offered cooked food. This dream was taken as a sign that her gastric condition (najam) was caused by spirit disturbance. The significance of this dream relates to the identification of spirits with wild animals as well as the opposition of the spirit world to the human world.

Two forms of pathogenic spirit affliction, pais-layu-layu and dawawa jalu, are recognized by the Taman. They differ from each other mainly in that the former includes spirit encounters in dreams and the latter involves meeting spirits in waking life. Characteristic of both syndromes is withdrawal, confusion, and a distaste for food. Particularly in adults, sexual fantasies and their disavowal are often at the root of these symptoms that do not cease upon being treated. It is possible that the diagnosis of these syndromes in children, with whom an element of sexual fantasy may be lacking, is based on an extension of these aspects of the condition in adults.

Pais Layu-Layu *(Pining-away illness)*

Pais layu-layu, the quintessential affliction of the prospective balien, is the retrospective reinterpretation of regular illness in light of a relevant dream. A single dream of sexual encounter with a beautiful person may be sufficient cause for a reevaluation of a person's symptomatology.

The term "pais layu-layu" itself means a sickness that comes and goes inexplicably. A characteristic of pais layu-layu is that after medical treatment the sufferer gets better temporarily, then relapses. The term "layu-layu" means "wilting, fading away, withering, weak, or drooping." "Pais layu-layu" can be translated as "pining-away illness." It is at first undefinable. A man who had recently undergone a mengadengi ceremony to treat this illness said, "While one is sick, one doesn't know what it is. For example, you can't eat, but you don't know what is wrong. But other people notice the difference."

Bolom explained that when she was first treated by baliens in the mengadengi ceremony, her original complaints were stomachache, vomiting, and nausea. She said she felt as if there were a baby inside her. Other symptoms included constipation, stomach cramps, and loss of appetite. Along with these symptoms she experienced dreams of seduction. In this context, her dreams of seduction were interpreted as indicative of spirit involvement. (In themselves, the sexual dreams may not have induced her to seek treatment.) What was unusual, her family members said, was that if she came across *kayu ara* (*Ficus sp.*) in the forest she could not pass because she would hear the voice of the man from her dream.

Another woman, Samarai, recalled that she had had realistic sexual dreams for three or four years but that another dream alerted her to the urgency of her sickness. In the dream she participated in the menyarung ceremony with other women, including her dead mother.

Generally, it is the longing for the person in the dreams that signals that they are part of a larger pattern of pais layu-layu. Most of the baliens interviewed indicated that they had experienced sexual dreams continually before initiation and felt a longing for the fantasized figure.

To some extent the influence of ghosts and spirits is deduced from the coexistence of sickness and a dream. For many of those who subsequently became baliens, the feeling of incapacity and malaise was not oppressive in itself. One informant said of pais layu-layu, "It is not so painful. You can still work, but you become thin and yellow. It is caused by being with a dead person." According to some people, another part of the pattern of those destined to become baliens is their sense of melancholia: they sometimes sit quietly, just pondering, and are sad for no reason.

A man chronicled his wife's pais layu-layu in the following narrative:

> Before she was initiated as a manang [balien] her sickness was ordinary, but she became thin, didn't want to eat, and dreamed of meeting a man who wanted to take her away; in the daytime she remembered him. She didn't want me anymore. She'd be in bed with me, and then say, "he has arrived." After she was initiated, these dreams never came again. [The spirits] had all been caught and turned into stones.

Dawawa Jalu (*Possession by a Being*)

Dawawa jalu is not a dream, nor is there necessarily an implication of sexual longing. Rather, it is a vision appearing to be a human being that is actually a ghost or other spirit. As a syndrome, dawawa jalu takes the form of a recurring apparition, usually accompanied by a person's ineluctable attraction to the vision. It is specifically a balien's sickness. Besides seeing a nonexistent person or persons, other symptoms are physical weakness and loss of appetite. Total immobility—a sudden inability to move or speak—is another sign of dawawa jalu. The primary distinction between dawawa jalu and pais layu-layu is that in the former the visions appear in waking life instead of or as well as in dreams.[2]

Most informants stated that sexual ideas were the most prominent symbol. However, a recently initiated balien, a thirty-eight-year-old divorcée with one child, told the following narrative:

> It wasn't that I wanted to become a manang, but when I walked in the forest I saw an imaginary person. This started two or three years ago. At first

I didn't believe it. Then I told my family. They said maybe there was a ghost or "being" (jalu). The "being" resembled a number of real people—my child, friends, male and female. After that, whenever I saw rice it looked like ants to me and I didn't want to eat it. I was afraid of vines, thinking they were snakes. I frequently fainted.

This balien mentioned apparitions seen in waking life but not dreams, specifically not erotic dreams. Despite the lack of explicit sexual content in this woman's narrative, it may be supposed that her symptoms disguise sexual issues (Bernstein 1993a; Fenichel 1945). Furthermore, she may have felt inhibited discussing this aspect of her visions. Generally, it was the husbands of female baliens who confided such details to me. The nature of the other symptoms suggests a hysterical syndrome that would include this sexual fantasy material.

In another case, a woman had been sick for three years. After fainting for the first time, she was treated by a public health worker who told her she had low blood pressure, but she did not get better from his treatment. She saw visions of a man who wanted to seduce her, an indication that her ailment was caused by dawawa jalu. People in the village said she would have to become a balien. Her sons wanted to have her treated in Serukam Hospital, hundreds of miles away, but they agreed to let her try this traditional cure first.

A male balien's story was also typical: "I did not know what sickness I had but was confused and saw [an apparition of] a girl. The girl was like a lover. It was usual for me to cry because I could not catch the spirit. When I was sick, I would notice that I had rattan cuts all over, but did not feel them, because a spirit had entered me." Another man who had been treated for dawawa jalu stated that he would faint if he encountered one of the apparitions of the three or four girls that were disturbing him.

Several baliens I interviewed said their preinitiatory illness was dawawa jalu rather than pais layu-layu. The family of one balien said that her dawawa jalu was sent by a spirit that resembled her husband. The first time she was sick, she fainted while just sitting. The woman herself could not be specific about the kind of spirit bothering her. She said only that she had seen it and that it took the form of a man, but that it never gave its name.

Yet another balien said that her sickness was not dawawa jalu but *dawawa tamang*: capture of the soul by her husband's spirit double, which had the same name as her husband and looked like him, "only better." She felt an uncontrollable love for this apparition and stated that her heart was always going to him.

Dawawa jalu conforms to what Douglass Price-Williams calls the "waking dream," strikingly realistic imaginary scenes over which the subject feels no sense of control. These waking dreams, unlike active imagination, "are usually spontaneous and characteristically burst into an individual's ordinary consciousness" (Price-Williams 1987: 251).

Spirit Disturbance

The illnesses dawawa jalu and pais layu-layu, which can be grouped togeth-er as spirit disturbance, are different from illnesses associated with spirit attack. The spirit that attacks a person does so generally out of revenge and is not visible to the victim. The prototypical concept of such an illness is badi or dabalas jalu, revenge for behavior that hurt the spirit. The spirit that disturbs a person presents the victim with an entire persona, however indis-tinct, in dreams and apparitions. Spirits are said to target their victims in spirit disturbance, but their motivation in these cases is morbid concupis-cence. They are able magically to overrun the minds of their beloved victims with thoughts of them. (Turner's [1968] term "affliction" seems an appro-priate characterization of these disturbances.) Such captivation is distinct from spirit attack, and it is also different from spirit possession and spirit mediumship, in which a person becomes a receptacle and mouthpiece for a spirit (see Firth 1967; Lewis 1971; Winzeler 1993).

The notion that the spirit who loves a person would seek to persecute that person is paradoxical. In the view of Anne Parsons (1969: 193), the delusion of victimization involves a "transformation of affect into belief," resulting from the rejection by the ego of a loved object. I have suggested elsewhere (Bernstein 1993a: 187), based on psychoanalytic writings, that some tabooed love object, possibly a parent, may be the underlying object of the fantasy in these illnesses of affliction.

As shown in Table 4.1, on page 64, illness by spirit disturbance (or affliction) is a separate category of illness distinct from spirit attack but it is also continuous with spirit attack and more serious than it within the same model of illness causation. Certain bodily illnesses generally attributed to spirit attack may be related to spirit affliction if they disappear and reappear in some pattern, and if there is a recurring relevant dream. Also, the treat-ment for spirit affliction is preceded by treatment for spirit attack. Finally, an advanced spirit seance, *menindoani* (see Chapter 6), is used instead of mengadengi in treating some illnesses labeled pais layu-layu, particularly if involvement from a spirit of the dead (*Antu Bangkai*) rather than a nature or animal spirit (sai) is suspected. Those people whose illnesses are resolved at this stage do not continue treatment by holding mengadengi, and they are not seen as destined to become baliens.

Needs Expressed Through Illness

In both pais-layu-layu and dawawa jalu, chronic disorders involving sense-less suffering begin to make sense subjectively when seen as the result of victimization. Pain and illness are associated with conflicts about desires projected onto a spirit realm, since it is denied that they originate in the sub-ject's own mind. In this regard, clinical findings about hysterical illnesses

(Nemiah 1988; Abse 1959; Krohn 1978; Fenichel 1945) and even the hysterical personality (Blacker and Tupin 1977; Shapiro 1965) are informative for purposes of comparison to the balien's predisposing condition.

Hysteria refers to psychoneurotic disorders that may include either dissociation (alteration in consciousness and personal identity) or conversion (somatic and sensory disturbances), or both. Psychoanalytic theory holds that the hysteric expresses repressed wishes first in fantasy and then in bodily symptoms. Clinical symptoms of hysteria include episodic disturbances in which "an ego-alien constellation of ideas and emotions occupies the field of consciousness" (Abse 1959: 274). Such ego-alien ideas and feelings may be interpreted as spirit involvement. In hysteria, symptoms indirectly communicate wants and needs when direct expression is difficult. In clinical cases of hysteria, as in the Taman folk syndromes, patients commonly attribute their outbursts not to their own feelings but to alien forces (Shapiro 1965: 128). The disturbances of appetite may also represent sexual or other conflicts (Fenichel 1945: 145–147).

Related to the concept of hysteria is the phenomenon of somatization, meaning that "problems of a psychological or social order are experienced through a somatic imagery of physical pain" (Wikan 1990: 176). Unni Wikan comments further about somatization, as it is used in Bali: "Indeed, interpersonal problems will find their way to a person's body and be expressed *through* it, for avenues for dealing with such problems in everyday life are strictly limited. In the Taman case, physical illness is often expressed as badet (najam in Malay), an illness affecting the gastrointestinal system that typically "travels" from one spot to another. This migratory aspect is often characteristic of psychogenic pain (see Shorter 1992).

Symptoms of illness may also be used unconsciously in imitation of the behavior of others, to express a desire to participate in the activities of the balien—to join the balien group as an initiate—a phenomenon called pathomimesis (Schwartz 1976). This does not necessarily mean that the people who suffer from these disturbances desire in any way to become healers. An interesting aspect of somatization, mentioned by Edward Shorter (1994: 140), is that throughout history people "have always tended to take on whatever psychosomatic symptoms were popular at the moment" within their milieu. Shorter documents the existence of "fashions" in the symptomatology of somatic complaints in European and U.S. history. Similarly for the Taman, symptoms have a sociocultural context. The balien system provides a socially acceptable and culturally meaningful way of repressing sexually disturbing material by projecting it onto a world of supernatural beings. The mengadengi ceremony is the social process of recognizing and coming to terms with these feelings, while menyarung (the initiation ceremony) is the process for curing the afflicted person by formally altering that person's status from that of a victim of spirits to one who has made peace with spirits. Successfully initiated baliens are, in effect, cured: Their delusions and somatic symptoms disappear, and they can harness their imaginative powers to benefit others. Previously sick and maladapted, they are now well adapted because of their integration in a specialized role. The transformation from patient (sick person) into healer (novice member of the thaumaturgical association of baliens) allows insight and resynthesis of thought processes, integration within society in a new role, and a way of dealing with threatening ego-alien sexual impulses.

Balien initiation involves a curious, even paradoxical, reversal in the relationship with spirits, in that spirits that have instigated illness and must be neutralized are accommodated and domesticated. As Lewis (1986: 89) has stated, "The spirit or spirits responsible for the initial (and retrospectively initiatory) trauma are subsequently transformed into 'helping spirits' by a process recalling that referred to by psychologists as 'identifying with the aggressor.'" As we shall see, the spirits neutralized in the stone-capturing ceremonies are indeed transformed.

The Balien's Destiny

Unconscious factors may propel a person into induction as a balien. But any person who admitted to such an aspiration or who was discovered to have become a balien voluntarily would be rejected as a fraud. The eager balien defies the dogma that authentic baliens acquire their vocation as the result of victimization. Not only is balien status not sought, but people avoid the prospect of becoming a balien even after they have been instructed that they must do so. The issue of choosing to become a balien is viewed instead as a matter of saving one's own life. Whether the treatment works and the person goes on to become an effective balien or the initiate does not recover, but sickens and dies, is considered in terms of fate and not the quality of the ceremony or the motivation of the initiate.

The decision to go through with the full initiation depends on the weighing of several factors:

1. The tips of the areca blossom that is cracked open at the conclusion of the mengadengi ceremony indicate by their morphology (straight or curled) whether the person is destined to become a balien.
2. If the symptoms predisposing a person to be treated by baliens subside and then recur after mengadengi, it means the person must continue with the process and become a balien. However, if the condition is unchanged after the mengadengi, it means that this is not the correct course. If symptoms do not recur, there is no urgency to proceed with the initiation, even if the areca blossom oracle indicates that it is necessary.
3. There may be positive and negative opinions within the family affecting a person's decision to become a balien candidate. In the cases ongoing during my fieldwork the issue was presented as a

question of old ways versus new ways. However, deeper interpersonal relationships are reflected in these cases. Once a consensus has been reached, the financial backing of the family is needed to support the large capital outlay required for the menyarung ceremony, since the candidate, who is sick, is usually unable to work at full capacity.

Social Pressure and Resistance

The prospect of becoming a balien has little appeal. The layout of capital for the ceremony is a major deterrent. The total expense of a *menyarung* ceremony was estimated by most people to be between Rp 150,000 and Rp 200,000—equivalent to a household's income for as much as six months. Because of the expense, the ceremony is commonly held following a harvest; only those who have other capital can afford to hold the ceremony at other times of the year.

Considering the effect of a menyarung ceremony on the family budget, it is understandable that all members of the household have an opinion on this matter. A male candidate said after his one-night mengadengi ceremony that the decision about whether to continue the process to full initiation depended on the consensus of his family. He said that if his wife and children preferred, he would become a balien, but that he himself did not want to do so. He would wait for the arrival of all of his children before making a decision. But he had apparently overruled the opinion of his teenaged daughters, who were embarrassed by the prospect. One daughter I talked to was a secondary school pupil in Putussibau, living in a Catholic dormitory and strongly oriented toward Catholicism.

> She was clearly embarrassed if not ashamed about the matter. She said he [her father] wanted to become a balien, and it was up to him and she would not advise otherwise, but he did not have to become a balien if whatever it was that was disturbing him—which she did not want to discuss—no longer disturbed him, and he was not sick anymore, so she saw no reason for him to want to do it, and thought it unnecessary.

From this case it appears that a person may actually be quite willing to become a balien despite protests to the contrary.

In another case a young woman was treated by baliens in a mengadengi at the insistence of her mother. During the ceremony she sat sullenly and refused the baliens' invitations to join the dancing. According to the oracle at the conclusion of the ceremony, she was destined to become a balien. She had no interest in becoming a balien but admitted that if her illness returned she would have no choice but to continue the treatment to the stage of initiation.

In a case that I did not witness, a girl about the age of puberty who was told she was destined to become a balien also refused invitations to dance.

She said at the time she could not become a balien and wanted to finish her education. (Her parents supported her in this; indeed, it is unheard of for a child to become a balien.) She was told to continue with the initiation when she reached adulthood. The girl's parents explained that if people are destined to become baliens, they cannot refuse, because if they do not undergo initiation, they can never be cured.

This belief was supported by the two baliens involved in the girl's case, who discussed between themselves the futility of avoiding the inescapable call to the balien's profession. They remembered how they had both tried to avoid becoming baliens by seeking cures from a Malay dukun. One abstained from eating pork for twelve years because it was a prohibition connected with the use of an amulet (jimat) she had been given by the dukun. In the end she threw out the amulet and became a balien because the spirit kept returning to disturb her. The other woman said that she kept a jimat in her mosquito net on orders of a dukun but that the spirit came in nonetheless. If a spirit targets a person ("has their address"), there is no way to keep it out, she said. So she discarded her jimat as well.

The *Menyarung* Ceremony

A person becomes a balien through a complex and expensive ceremony called menyarung. The name of this ceremony seems to derive from the term for a large circular sun hat (*sarung*) made from palm leaves. Such a hat (*sarung ase*), specially decorated with rice panicles, various leaves, flowers, and a kind of fish, is worn in the menyarung.[3] The ceremony lasts for three nights and days and, following a rest period of a night and a day, continues for another night and ends the following day. The main activities in this ceremony are chanting to spirits, inviting them to partake in the food being offered; dancing; "capturing" spirits (including those causing the disturbance), thereby turning them to stone; and "piercing" the candidate's fingertips and eyes.

The menyarung ceremony takes place at the house or longhouse apartment of the candidate. If the candidate lives in a small longhouse apartment, one or more walls may be taken down to make more space. If the house is not sufficient to hold the many guests, a kinsman's house may be used for the purpose. During the ceremony, the candidate sits inside a small space underneath an offering structure, *kalangkang,* that is filled with food offerings, draped with a cloth, and suspended from a ceiling rafter with a cord. Long leaves are hung around the sides of the kalangkang, with the effect of enclosing the interior space like a cubicle.

The ceremony must be well planned and organized. Many materials, such as various kinds of leaves and fishes, need to be assembled. The acquisition of many of these may be problematic, particularly on short notice, but menyarung may not proceed unless the complete set of materials, objects,

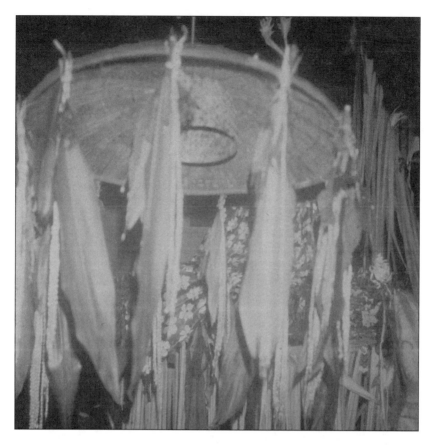

Sarung ase (rice hat worn in menyarung ceremony).

and ingredients has been assembled. It is said that if the kalangkang is not full, the spirits will not come near. Besides the kalangkang itself, many items need to be made, including a uniform for the candidate (if a woman). At least seven baliens, including one male balien, must be contracted for the duration of the five-day ceremony. (The ceremony may not be held with a total of seven participants including the candidate, since that is thought to bring misfortune, the number seven being associated with death.) More than 200 pounds of rice is needed just for payment of the baliens. A substantial volume of liquor is also required for the baliens' consumption during the ceremony. Participants and a large number of spectators must also be fed for the duration of the ceremony. It is expected that virtually everyone from the village or longhouse will attend at least briefly, and guests from throughout the village complex will be welcomed. At times 100 people may be present during the menyarung ceremony.

The existence of a large audience for any menyarung ceremony suggests that it is a performance, analogous to the presentation of a drama.[4] While certain members of the audience assist with the ceremony, most do not, yet their presence is required and serves a number of essential functions. The spectators serve as an audience to appreciate and respond to the artistic and humorous aspects of the ceremony. Artistry occurs in dancing, chanting, and regalia; all are traditional and highly regarded forms of expression. The baliens are as if onstage, and in this regard their work would be wasted if not enacted before an audience. The members of the audience serve not merely as spectators but as witnesses. By receiving the messages of the ritual and by simply providing their presence, they enable the ceremony to have an efficacy it would not have otherwise.[5] The capture of the stones, a public spectacle, is authenticated by being witnessed by the audience, thereby legitimizing both the explanation of the illness as being from spirits and the efficacy of the cure through spirit capture (petrification). The audience also witnesses the areca blossom augury, which validates the effectiveness of the ceremony. By adding to the overall number present, audience members serve the hosts by increasing the event's "ritual involution" (Tambiah 1985: 153).

Unlike the audience at a theatrical performance or sports event the people in attendance are guests, and must be treated with hospitality to the best of the hosts' abilities. Food and refreshments must be provided: minimally, rice and dried fish at mealtimes, and sweet coffee during breaks in the ceremony.

Scheduling and Preparation

After a decision has been made to hold a menyarung ceremony and the necessary capital has been accumulated, at least seven baliens (including at least one male) must be contracted for the five-day period. In scheduling the ceremony, custom must be respected: If a person in the village is seriously ill, or if there is a state of ritual prohibition (buling) following death, there are objections to the ceremony because the noise it generates is disrespectful. In one case, a family holding a menyarung ceremony paid the family holding buling the full fine, Rp 6,000, beforehand so that they could feel free to make as much noise as they wanted. However, if a person has just died, the ceremony must be postponed because of the danger from ghosts in the vicinity.

Efforts are made to wait until all interested persons can attend, especially the beneficiary's children living in distant places, so that they can help with the considerable work. While the members of the beneficiary's kindred obtain the necessary materials for the kalangkang, the baliens contracted to perform the ceremony do most of the work preparing the kalangkang and decorating it. This work takes several hours.

A *baju kalawat,* the special embroidered blouse unique to the female balien, must be prepared. (In one case, a family had commissioned several baliens to make the blouse, paying them each Rp 2,000 per day in addition to supplying the materials.) A long bead on a twine string is also prepared to be worn by the initiate around the torso for some months after the inauguration. Besides the blouses, the female baliens wear fancy batik skirts, and the male baliens wear dress shirts during the ceremony.[6] All the baliens wear a headdress (*tikolo'*) decorated with flowers, shaved wood, and strings of cubed coconut meat.

During the three-day-long ceremony, several different uniforms are worn. The baliens change their dress several times, usually putting on their finest clothes before the night service.[7] Women usually wear the baju kalawat; however, not all clothes worn in the ceremony are formal, and baliens may wear T-shirts at times.

Another important piece of equipment in the menyarung ceremony is a bamboo pole split open at the top, tied with a cloth to a ceiling rafter and extending to the ground. This pole, called *buluh ayu* (decorated bamboo), is grasped by the balien while singing the chant, to contact the spirit world and broadcast the song. It faces eastward—the direction in which the sun rises, which is associated with the direction of the living.[8]

In part, the baliens' preparations are intended to make them impervious to spirits. At the beginning of the ceremony, baliens wear cloths folded in squares over their heads to prevent spirits from affecting them. They also cover their bodies with an oil (*polek mo*) that enables them both to see spirits and to make them invisible to spirits.

The Invitation and Capture of Spirits

One balien acts as the leader by grasping the buluh ayu and leading chants. The first chant is made to Piang (Grandmother) Siunsun Amas, the goddess of the baliens, beseeching her to bless the participants, the kalangkang, the offerings, the house in which the ceremony is held, and the land on both sides of the river. Finally, the candidate is blessed. The leader sings a short phrase, and the rest of the baliens sing the chorus by repeating the last word or several syllables of each stanza (see Appendix E). The baliens' chants (*timang*) are not sung in the standard Taman language but in an archaic (*jolo*) dialect specific to these particular chants. This language is not understandable to most laymen, and some people say it is not a human language but rather the language of spirits and ghosts.

Following the chanting, music lasting for several minutes is played by some members of the audience (mainly girls) on chinaware bowls, drums, and small gongs. A second chant, *timang malong sai* (chant to call the spirits), is delivered in the same manner as the first chant. Spirits are called in the order of the "villages" (locations in the forest or river) they inhabit,

beginning with the farthest upstream and ending with the farthest downstream. The headman of each village or longhouse in the spirit world is
invited, and all the spirits, male and female, are asked to come without
exception. Here is a brief excerpt of such a chant:[9]

> Grandmother kalangkang.
> Enter the house.
> See the kalangkang used for X this night.
> Let us see the kalangkang together.
> You are all called.
> Thus I call you.
> Previously I received you in the kalangkang.
> It won't even take the whole night.
> Not everyone from upstream has arrived yet.
> The river with spirits that are called, from Sala' Anyut they are called.
> From every longhouse.
> Enter in X's house.
> Our appointment has arrived, it is only three nights.
> Gather from Awain River. [a river far upstream of the village in which
> this ceremony was performed]
> Males and females, all descend.
> From Taigin Babak River.
> From Nanga Bunut.
> From Buling Saung.
> From Ulu Pinangnin.
> From Luat Lam Ulu Batu.
> Come downstream.
> Jamilu [name of a spirit].
> Sanan Kalamit.
> Pasa' Olo'.
> Manjungen.
> Come without exception.

Following this chant, percussion music starts again. When a good
rhythm has been established, the baliens arise and the candidate joins them
in forming a queue.[10] The leader of the chant is at the head of this queue, and
the candidate is somewhere in the middle; the order remains the same
throughout the ceremony. A woman serves them beverages from a kettle:
usually palm wine or rice wine, though coffee may also be served in the
morning. The baliens then walk around the kalangkang, soon breaking into
a dance that continues for up to twenty minutes. Like the chant, dance is
used to summon spirits.

The dance is then repeated, signifying the arrival of spirits. During the
second dance the baliens pick up bundles of suri, *taraksio* (*Tetractomia obovata*), and *banoh* (*Gendarussa vulgaris*) leaves in one hand and bowls in the
other. (At times the leaf bundles are worn by the baliens at the back of the
hair like a bonnet.) Each of the baliens then sees a spirit and "catches" (*paut*)
it by gently tapping the leaves on the rim of a bowl, producing a stone. As
soon as this happens, assistants (family members or affines of the

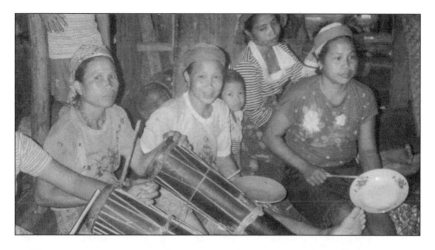

The percussion section at the menyarung ceremony is dominated by girls.

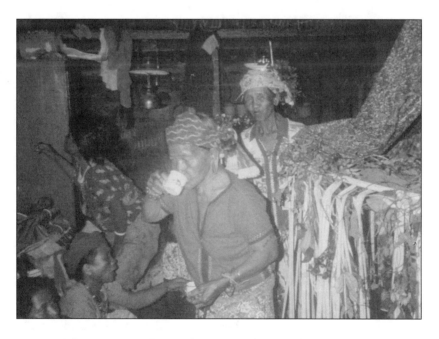

Baliens are served cups of marem (palm wine) before dancing.

candidate) with bottles of cooking oil rush to sprinkle oil on the stones to harden them, while the baliens feel the stones. The baliens then place the bowls containing the stones on their heads and rejoin the circle, dancing with the stones, before putting the bowls down and sitting in place on the

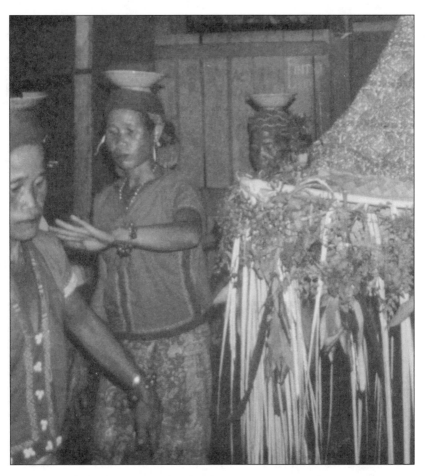

Baliens dance around kalangkang in menyarung ceremony.
On their heads are bowls containing stones they have just caught.

floor again. The stones are displayed in an arc, giving the audience a chance
to see which stones have been collected. (No audience member may touch
them.) The stones are then gathered into a larger container, and after a recess
the process begins again.

This sequence is performed three times at night and three times during
the day, for three days. The candidate participates in the dances but does not
have leaves or a bowl and does not catch a stone until the final night, when
the spirit that has been disturbing him or her is caught. After one day of rest,
there is a reprise starting the subsequent night and ending the following day,
called *ium babari.*

The Insertion of Hooks

During the second night of the ceremony, the candidate's fingertips and eyes are supposed to be pierced with metal hooks (*rabe* or *kait*) similar to fishing hooks. As music is being played, the baliens enter the kalangkang, where the candidate is reclining. They huddle around the candidate and fan him or her with their leaf bundles. What happens next is not visible from outside the kalangkang, but according to the custom, the baliens put the fishing hooks into both tips of the candidate's middle fingers. To do this, the hook is first dipped in the medicinal herb *tantamu* and then pushed into the flesh with a stone. Next, another fishing hook is used to cut the outer tissue (perialimbic sclera) of the eyeballs. The baliens then rub the candidate's body with their stones, using the bubut technique (see Chapter 6) to remove all disease objects.

I have heard from nonbaliens that these procedures do not hurt and that they cause neither bleeding nor scars. I have never seen scars on the fingertips of baliens that would indicate that such a procedure had been performed. One balien told me that if this were done to anyone but a balien, it would cause bleeding. But another balien I interviewed contradicted that, saying that the operation does cause bleeding and long-lasting pain. "How could it not hurt?" she asked rhetorically. A nonbalien said that the piercing of both the fingers and the eyes did in fact take place and that the incisions caused pains lasting seven or eight days. I have also been told that a balien's fingers rubbed over a patient feel scratchy to the patient.

The initiatory meaning and symbolism of hooks and piercing in the menyarung ceremony is discussed fully later, but it is worthwhile to raise the question of whether piercing is or can possibly be real. Since I have never seen any evidence of scars, bleeding, or mutilation, I do not believe that the flesh or eyeballs of initiates are actually pierced, much less that metal hooks are embedded in them. However, it is possible that actual hooks are used and that they perhaps touch, scratch, or even puncture body parts, and I have no evidence that absolutely nothing is done to the candidate. It is even possible for medically untrained practitioners to cut the perialimbic sclera without damaging the eye, since it is known that untrained healers in medieval Europe performed such surgery to remove cataracts (Vincent Sanchez, personal communication). Still, it is probably more realistic to assume that baliens are not pierced but that everyone in the society either thinks that they are or else deliberately perpetuates the myth of the pierced balien.

Serious and Amusing Performances

Whereas the second night of the ceremony is characterized in part by highly serious behavior and dramatization, other events of the night have the effect of light entertainment. On that night a "boat stone" (*Batu Paru*) is caught during a mock fishing expedition. The mood of the ceremony changes as the baliens use poles to simulate propelling a canoe through shallow water and catch people's sandals and other objects on their fishing poles. This portrayal of a fishing expedition and the interaction with the audience evince a humorous mode, with the baliens taking the roles of actors and comedians.

The third night of the menyarung ceremony is the climax, when the baliens imitate the actions of individual animal spirits and catch the most important stones. These stones have special purposes, and special procedures must be followed in order to obtain them. In catching them, the baliens embody spirits, whose arrival is represented by the stereotyped behavior of the baliens.[11] (One balien described the feeling on being possessed by the deer spirit: "A deer with horns takes your soul and eats grass. It is as if someone grabbed your leg and took you on a trip.") On the arrival of Antu Anak, the baliens eat boiled eggs; this is symbolic of Antu Anak's predilection for eating men's testicles (eggs being an explicit metaphor for testicles). They go around the audience, offering bits of egg to each person, almost forcing people to eat them. This adds to the menyarung's sense of wildness, humor, and absurdity, but like every other element, it has a serious purpose: to ensure that the people in the audience do not fall victim to the dangers of kempunan (see Chapter 4).

These are some animal spirit stones, and the procedures or phenomena associated with their capture.

Batu Bau (eagle stone).   The offering required for catching this stone is a boiled chicken that is hung up.

Batu Sit Bara (a kind of bird stone).   This spirit makes a distinctive sound if it arrives.

Batu Payoh (deer stone).   If this spirit arrives, it likes to drink saltwater. When dancing, the baliens eat *riribu* (*Lygodium flexuosum*) and *kalambibit* (*Merremia umbellata*) vines and claw downward, in inviting or being possessed by this spirit.

Batu Baruang (bear stone).   Its arrival is presaged by the baliens' hand movements during the dance, a downward clawing motion.

Batu Induayo (a female spirit).   Its arrival is indicated by baliens waving their hands backwards over their shoulders while dancing. (Possibly in imitation of the pendulous breasts of Induayo, which must be dragged in this way.) The stone is pockmarked.

Batu Antu Anak (a male spirit).   The baliens grasp upward, eat eggs, giggle, make screeching noises, and make the characteristic sound of *Antu Anak*: "kik kik kik."

Other stones of animal spirits that may be collected at this time are *Batu Lalawi* or *Batu Labi-Labi* (tortoise stone), *Batu Pari-Pari* (ray fish stone), *Batu Harimau* (tiger stone), and *Batu Tangkiling* (pangolin stone). Not every balien possesses a complete assemblage of stones, and a balien may possess certain *Batu Kait* that no one else has.

Along with the stones captured at the menyarung ceremony, a tiny fleck or pebble (*ansan*) is caught. Like the other stones, it is an essential part of the balien's equipment, but its purpose is different: It is later put into a vial of coconut oil to become *polek mo,* the "medicine" that baliens rubs over their arms, face, and equipment (*pangait*—see Chapter 6) before beginning work, to help them see the spirits and simultaneously make their own bodies invisible to the spirits. This charm is important because it fortifies the balien's power needed to manipulate spirits. When this fleck is caught, oil is sprinkled on it and all the baliens look at it. It is put into a small glass vial. The baliens mix the pebble medicine with each of their own bottles of polek mo, pooling their own medicine with that of the novice. Along with the stones, this bottle is given to the initiate, who ties it with cord to a basket containing his or her stones.

On the third night the candidate must catch the offending spirit responsible for the affliction. Because of the power of the wild spirit, the candidate may faint at this juncture. (This happened to a man who attempted during the mengadengi service to catch the spirit that had disturbed him: He grabbed her the wrong way, and she punched him, knocking him unconscious.) The baliens also symbolically attack the initiate and one another. In this performance, people collapse and are revived. This display is a drama portraying death, contact with the souls of the dead, and rebirth. The following is a description of this part of the ceremony.

> The baliens hold two suri leaves, one in each hand, but they sit down again without having caught stones. The candidate appears to get in a brawl, collapses, is brushed with a leaf by one balien, who says something over her, and is covered with a cloth by another. Now she is brushed with a bunch of other leaves, and is revived. Now three baliens attack the male balien the same way, and he collapses. They are laughing. They drag him to the other side of the room. One balien brushes his head with the leaves, the others scurry back to their places.
>
> The music stops and everything calms down. The man jokes, everything is okay, and a group of other women laugh. One is laughing uncontrollably at a joke he made about dried fish.

During the next day of this ceremony, there was another ritualized attack on the initiate.

The baliens "stab" the initiate with leaves and she collapses. She's down. The leader brushes her body. Her head is covered. Now the bunch of wet leaves is patted on her head, and the leader blows on her head or into her ear to revive her. She puts the headband [beaded with cubes of coconut] back on the initiate's head. The initiate stands here for a while then rejoins the procession. Some of the baliens pick up leaves again. Others are sitting down. One of them attacks the male balien and he collapses. Now she attacks all the others; they are cracking up laughing. They all must be patted on the head with the wet bunch of leaves to be revived. Actually, some of them seem to get back up without any help. Everyone is seated, and the music stops.

These actions, like other parts of the ceremony, are said to be determined "by the stones," namely, by the spirits that arrive and possess the participants. The baliens are highly suggestible to each other's behavior and to the roles of the spirits being invoked. For example, a story was told of a boy in the audience at one menyarung ceremony who made the sound of Antu Anak while the baliens were dancing. Upon hearing this sound, a balien in the midst of dancing lunged at him, tore his clothes, and tried to claw his eyes and testicles, a behavior identified with Antu Anak. To prevent the balien from killing the boy, another person gave her a raw chicken, which she ate whole, feathers and all.

Some humorous, playful, or aggressive behavior by the participants may simply represent the baliens' playing up to the audience (the great majority of whom consist of children) for entertainment. For example, while dancing, some baliens tend to prance exaggeratedly. I observed baliens drinking liquid from a vat and spitting it at the audience. At another ceremony, people in the audience suspended a rope that the baliens, dancing in a row, had to jump over when they reached it. Another crowd was delighted when a youth, using obscene language, taunted a balien. The audience is unruly but does not seriously interfere with the ceremony.

Some humorous behavior by the baliens appears to be ritualized, such as begging for cigarettes (even pulling them out of the mouths of spectators) and sucking at them while giggling. Smoking—especially smoking commercially manufactured cigarettes—is uncommon among Taman women, and in most of Indonesia outside the metropolis, smoking is considered unfeminine, but the baliens make a fuss about smoking cigarettes at a certain point in the ceremony.

The distinctive humor of the menyarung ceremony consists in the baliens' performing wild and ludicrous forms of behavior and sometimes engaging members of the audience. Terence Turner (1977) has attempted to explain humor in ritual as resulting from the formal structure of ritual itself. In Turner's structural model of social transitions in rites of passage, a person's move from a lower level in a hierarchy to a higher one is a "transformational operation."

The actor has in effect shifted from one set of role categories, in which he played certain roles towards other actors occupying a complementary set of role categories, to become himself an occupant of the complementary set of role categories, playing the same roles towards others as were played to him by others when he occupied the first set of roles. The actor has, from his point of view, inverted the pattern of role relations defined by the matrix. (Turner 1977: 56)

It is the transition from the lower level to the higher one (the "liminal phase") that is characterized by humor and wildness. In Turner's view,

it is [the] hierarchical relation between the liminal phase [which expresses transcendent and transformational principles] and the profane social states or categories that form the terminal points of the ritual process which in turn accounts for the peculiar properties of the rites associated with this phase. The inverted, paradoxical, "anti-structural" qualities of these rites are precisely the sort which characterize the relationship of a higher level to a lower level (from the point of view of the latter). (Turner 1977: 68)

The menyarung ceremony, as an initiation ceremony, may be likened to the rites of passage being considered by Turner (following Van Gennep 1960; see also V. Turner 1967, 1969). Even though admission to the ranks of the balien is not a generalized change in status akin to that in a puberty ceremony, it is characterized by an inversion of the binary role from patient to healer. Therefore, it is understandable that wildness and disorder (an inversion of the solemnity of ritual), not found in other balien ceremonies, occurs here.

Finding comedic elements in Sinhalese exorcism ceremonies (which are not initiatory), Kapferer (1977, 1991) accounts for them also in terms of the overall structure of the performance. For Kapferer, comedy requires internal inconsistency, in contrast to the "serious" parts of ritual (prior to the introduction of comedy), that are based on consistency. In addition, the effectiveness of comedy depends on the suspension of belief, a "play frame" that negates the attitude of belief and acceptance underlying the preceding serious ritual. Comedy occurs when the ritual performers break out of their role of executing a rite by interacting with or at least playing to the audience.

Concluding Phase

On the last day of the ceremony, the baliens all dance with the sarung ase (rice hat), an object from which, I hypothesize, the menyarung ceremony derives its name. If this hypothesis is correct, the sarung ase is of central importance in the ceremony. As the dancers circle the kalangkang, singing and dancing simultaneously, the hat is passed back to the dancer following in the queue until the candidate is wearing it. At this point, all the dancers leave the house (this is the first time the initiate has left the house since the start of the ceremony) to plant a small grove of plants, each of which has an important role in the balien's work. If the areca palms planted in this grove mature and become fruitful, it is taken as a sign, along with the cracked areca blossom augury, that the novice will go on to cure many people. The baliens then enter a boat that must make a circle in the river three times; afterward they return to the house to continue dancing. Musicians accompany the baliens throughout this stage of the ceremony. Others remain at the house, maintaining a percussion rhythm all the while.

All the baliens must drink pure tantamu juice at this time to purify their bodies. (Tantamu is the main medicinal herb used by the balien.) The juice has an extremely bitter taste, and it is said to make "regular" people sick. When I observed the drinking of tantamu, the baliens imbibed it with gusto.

After a one-day recess, the participants reconvene for a one-night continuation of the ceremony, ium babari, during which more stones are caught. The newly initiated balien wears a bead strung around her or his body for several months and is prohibited to eat certain foods. For eight days the meat of slaughtered animals is prohibited, and for three years certain fish (*joan, bantuh,* and *sare*) are also disallowed.

Areca Blossom Augury

On the third day of the menyarung ceremony, an augury is made by splitting open an areca blossom (*mayang pinang*) to determine whether the candidate has been cured and is destined to become a balien. The unopened blossom is kept in the upper tray of the kalangkang until the final night, when the baliens use it in a dance, passing it back from one dancer to the next. After all have danced with the blossom, it is given to the leading balien, who addresses the spirits of the ancestral (deceased) baliens in a chant while rubbing rice soaked in tantamu on the blossom.[12] The ancestral baliens are beseeched to give a sign of the candidate's destiny by ensuring that when it is opened all the tips of the blossom are curled (hook shaped); the blossom tips are ordered to be straight if the person is not fated to become a balien. The souls of the deceased baliens are called to witness the augury together with everyone present. These baliens of the past are believed to determine the outcome and are implored not to lie. The balien then counts to seven and cracks open the blossom with her hands. It is examined first by the baliens and then by other interested parties and people in the audience, who discuss the condition of the tips. After everyone has looked at it, it is hung up on the wall as a reminder of the outcome of the ceremony. There it remains in perpetuity, along with other artifacts of the menyarung ceremony, such as the kalangkang and the sarung ase.

In each of the ceremonies I witnessed, and in others that were described to me, the augury was interpreted to mean that the ceremony was appropriate and the person would become a balien. In one case I observed, a blossom intended for the ceremony was discarded at the last minute because it was

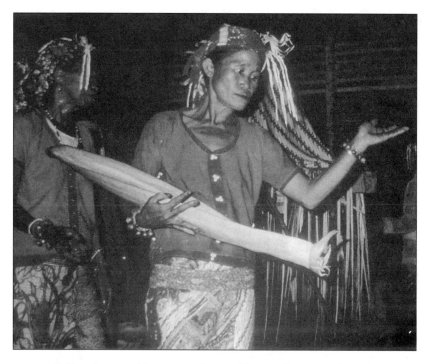

Balien dances with unopened areca blossom (mayang pinang).

noticed that it was slightly open and therefore defective; two men had to cut down another one. However, in another case, when the blossom was opened none of the tips appeared to be hooked except for a single strand in the middle. At the time it was said that the blossom was too young but that it was a good augury. I was told that just the strands in the front middle of the blossom represent the patient or candidate. The strands in the left side represent the participating baliens, and those in the right side represent unknown others (possibly the people in the audience). Later, when the patient's illness returned and other kinds of treatment were being considered, one balien who had participated in the ceremony admitted that the tips were straight.

The hooked tip of the blossom is taken as sign that the ancestral baliens have blessed the candidate's venture to become a balien. This form is emblematic because it reiterates the shape of the hook used to pierce the fingertips and the outer tissue of the candidate's eyes.

Payments

In payment for their service all the baliens (including the inductee) receive a portion of the rice used in the ceremony; informants estimated each balien's yield at about 25 to 30 pounds. Each balien also receives a chicken, ten bamboo tubes containing glutinous rice, a cup of sago flour (*sensagun*), one plate, and one knife. The leader of the chant receives a ceramic jar in addition to the other payments.

In a sense, the payment to the initate is not a real expense to the family putting on the ceremony, but it is revealing of the Taman attitude to custom that the honorarium must be paid, albeit within the family unit. (Likewise, other adat payments, although remaining within the family, must be paid if required.) The payment signifies the newly created status of the initiate who contracted the ceremony.

The payments or honoraria must be viewed as tokens rather than a true reimbursement for labor. Although the total expense to the family contracting the service is weighty, the revenue to the individual balien is paltry considering that she or he has worked for four days and nights, expending vast physical and psychic energy. While the monetary equivalents for marriages and torts in Taman adat law have been adjusted to keep pace with inflation, there are no standard equivalents to the balien's honorarium, which is defined in relatively inexpensive tokens; nor is the balien's share of rice fixed in terms of an absolute quantity.[13]

After the ceremony the initiate must pay his or her spouse half the marriage payment, in accordance with customary law, to compensate for the violation of the marriage caused by the sexual liaison with the spirit. Even though the initiate is an unwilling participant with a spirit partner, the relationship is still culpable, and the spirit seducer cannot of course be tried or forced to pay a fine.

Stones: Their Genesis, Transformation, and Meaning

Stones come into being in the menyarung ceremony, and it is through this event that the candidate's transformation from a sick person (patient) into a balien is effected. For baliens, stones define the contours of their profession and their entire way of life. Beyond the balien domain, stones, beads, and petrification are major themes in many Taman myths and legends. The important relationship each balien has with his or her stones epitomizes a more general cultural preoccupation.

Petrification is often a retribution for transgression, similar to the fate of Lot's wife in the Biblical parable. Harrisson (1965: 270–271) relates the story of Batu Indai Punga, in which an incestuous couple (mother and son) are struck by lightning and turned to stone. The following day several elders dream that the stone into which they had been transformed is a love charm. Harrisson (1965: 329–333) also mentions the legend of Batu Rabon, in the Lunsa vicinity, in which "all those who make fun of animals also make gods angry and thus they change the people into stones" (1965: 329). Dogs and cats had been dressed up in clothing and laughed at, breaking a taboo and thereby instigating this cataclysmic retribution.

Useful stones are said to originate from dreams. People dream of meeting stones that tell them of their usefulness.[14] One of my informants said, "In dreams an old person will tell you, 'here is a stone, you must feed it, and it will help you.'" Encountering strange stones is considered good fortune. The person who finds a *Batu Karuwe* (guardian stone) dreams the following night that the stone speaks to him and instructs him to "feed" it rice, glutinous rice, palm wine, and rice wine to ensure harvests of 1,000 gantangs of rice. These guardian stones are passed down. They can protect a person from danger when traveling: One man told me such a stone helped his son stay out of jail when he was captured as an illegal alien in Brunei.

Baliens' stones undergo a remarkable transformation from being pathogenic spirits that have tormented the victim. Petrified and neutralized by being tapped by leaves, they remain powerful and can now help the novice balien. Some balien stones take on additional identities, either as specific Batu Kait representing various animal and other spirits or as doubles, called *tamang,* representing the balien or his or her family members. Interestingly, these tamang do not have the same names as the balien; instead, they have distinct names, often with seemingly whimsical regal, archaic, or honorific airs. Thus, the stones are equated with some personal essence separate from the person's name. The names and identities are revealed to the novice balien by the stones in dreams. Through this process the balien gains insight into his or her new identity and is able to harness the power of the stones. The transformation is mutual: Through the process of a balien's stones being attributed with meanings, healing powers, and individual identities, the balien is transformed. This process begins after the mengadengi ceremony. Some of the stones collected in this ceremony may reveal their identities in dreams.

Essential to a balien's equipment are a complete set of tamang representing himself or herself and each living member of the household, as well as the grown children who have left the household and their spouses and children. No stones represent family members already dead at the time the stones are acquired. (Regrettably, I have no information on what becomes of a stone following the death of the person represented.) The collection of tamang stones corresponds to a broad cross-section of a balien's personal kindred and may be said to constitute a sort of psychological kindred. The baliens personify the stones, claiming that the stones talk to them and eat food and drink liquor. In chants baliens address their own stones and the stones of other baliens by name. In one case, a balien had lost a kit containing five stones, including her own tamang, when her canoe capsized. Her illness returned and she was forced to be reinitiated. During the ceremony she sang mournfully about how much she missed her "friends"—the stones. The new stones caught in the ceremony were given the same names as the ones she had lost.

In the Taman village of Melapi, in the early 1970s, all the baliens threw their stones into the Kapuas River when the whole village was converted to Catholicism. This prompted the relapse of the baliens' illnesses, and they all were reinitiated. This incident was interpreted as proof that the ways of the balien could not be eliminated. Being a balien is the inescapable solution to the metaphysical illnesses of dawawa jalu and pais layu-layu, and one cannot be a balien without stones.

Baliens' stones are not considered ordinary stones from the river (Batu Karangan) but are said to be lighter in weight than ordinary stones and are purportedly soft and wet when caught.[15] The cooking oil with which they are anointed when they are caught, making them a gleaming black, is supposed to harden them. It is said that baliens' stones are frightened away by ordinary stones: The spirits are afraid to descend if Batu Karangan are on the premises, and the baliens' stones disappear if placed together with ordinary stones. This conviction seems to contain an implicit warning to those who might attempt to introduce natural stones in a balien ceremony.

It is always amazing to see baliens produce huge rocks apparently from thin air. When dancing, they sometimes catch stones directly over the head of an audience member or in another manner that calls attention to the fact that the stones are not kept under their blouses or skirts. During one mengadengi ceremony, I overheard a balien say to her colleague, "We have already caught the male stones, now let's get the female stones." I have never seen how baliens hide their stones during ceremonies, but I did once inadvertently find two stones concealed inside a balien's purse that she later "caught" during the ceremony. Since many kinds of stones need to be acquired in a menyarung ceremony, it raises the question of whether baliens plan who will bring which stones.

The Taman believe in the reality of balien stones, and anyone who knew their secrets kept quiet about them to me. All Taman with whom I discussed the matter, whatever their opinion of the effectiveness of the baliens' cures, believed without question that the stones were of spirit origin and contradicted all suggestions that baliens obtained their stones from the river. I was once told that if a balien was ever seen collecting stones in the river, he or she would be fined and would never be trusted again.

The stones as used in the balien institution condense a view of human nature. They are seen literally as doubles of individual persons, comparable but hardly identical to the double (doppelgänger) in European literature and philosophy (Rank 1971). The Taman concept of stones as the doubles of humans provides substantial insight into their views on the soul and human nature. For example, their utility in enabling the balien's soul travel in seances (see Chapter 6) is based on the premise of the multiplicity and separability of souls and suggests that tamang stones are also thought to contain such souls capable of traveling outside the confines of the stone itself (see King 1975).

The manner in which spirits leave the stones therefore is related to the idea of the flight of the balien's soul and shows the special relationship between a balien and the stones. They are literally projections of the balien's own soul. The balien's intimate relationship with his or her stones may be compared to a girl's relationship to her dolls. A girl will project or represent aspects of herself onto her various dolls, relating to each of them different-ly. Like dolls, the stones are treated as if they were part of the human realm; they are talked and listened to, fed, and cared for.

In all, more than 100 stones are gathered in the menyarung and men-gadengi ceremonies, all devolving on the initiate. Many of these stones are unusual in shape. Long stones are petrifications of male spirits, while round ones are females. Even though the subject of the ceremony is haunted by one spirit, or at most by several spirits of the opposite sex, an entire range of stones of both sexes is collected at the menyarung ceremony.

The balien's stones are a dominant symbol, which, as Turner (1967) has defined the term, has multivocal and contradictory meanings. They are potent and alive but paralyzed. They have magical power for the balien, who has an intimate relationship with them, including a representation of identi-ty with one and a kinship relationship with others. The power of these stones cannot be activated by laymen.

The symbolic meaning of stones as exchanges for people is compre-hensible in that the balien's craft as a folk-medical discipline is about human values and the manipulation of human nature. The solidification of the spir-its represents the expected recovery of the disturbed person. The power of these stones can be used to cure others, to summon free spirits, and to carry the soul of the balien and bring the patient's soul to safety. But while the balien using stones is possessed or inspired by the power of stones, that power is perceived as being external to the balien's own self (De Vos 1990: chap. 2).

Hooks as Emblems

If stones are the dominant symbol of the balien's profession, then hooks are its emblems, following Raymond Firth's (1973) criterion that the sign shows no direct relation to the signified object but is related instead by an associa-tion of ideas. The hook motif is reflexive, reverberating through all phases of the balien's activities and evoking complex meanings specific to the balien's domain. The appearance of the hook motif in various phases of balienism reinforces the density of this symbol and provides a conceptual center of gravity to balienism as a cultural institution.

All informants suggested that they considered piercing an actual event, not merely a symbolic one.[16] One balien claimed that she could tell from a sensation in her fingertips that people were waiting at her house for treatment. It is said that if the fingertips have not been pierced with rabe (hooks), it is impossible to use the stones or perform any of the balien's work. Without the cut in the eye with a hook, it is likewise impossible to see the spirits. Piercing occurs before the candidate catches the spirit causing the disturbance. It may be argued that this piercing enables the novice to catch the stones and is the single most transforming action in the entire menyarung process.

The piercing of the eyes and fingertips of the initiate—whether it is actual or simply mimicked—pertain to the authenticity of the balien. Notwithstanding cross-cultural variation and the known effects of belief and altered states of consciousness in the experience and physiology of pain, it seems likely that actual piercing would involve pain and physical mutilation. A person seeking to become a balien for spurious reasons would probably be dissuaded from doing so because of the eventuality of enduring these initiations. Thus, the performance of piercing adds to the dogma of the involuntary nature of the balien's destiny. The initiation ceremony authenticates the baliens as a unique class of people.

The induction of pain in initiation rites is frequently an end with the purpose of transforming individual consciousness and bringing it under group control (Morinis 1985). The concept of piercing the eyeballs and fingertips during an initiation ceremony suggests that those parts of the body that are the major sensory organs for perceiving the external world are altered and disciplined for the specialized purpose of healing.

The Transformation of Identity

The balien's agenda is often characterized as being the work of spirits, inscrutable to the layman. While the layman has a conventional understanding of the spirit world, only the balien has a working relationship with the spirits. Having been cured of disturbances by being initiated into the group, the balien, more than anyone else in the society, is committed to a belief in the balien system of cures. Others may maintain a certain skepticism toward the balien's work—"half belief" as one Taman girl put it—but a balien believes in the reality of this system as no outsider can. Through initiation and the practice of cures, the novice is finally cured and experiences a conversion of belief and identity.[17]

This transformation of identity does not end at the conclusion of the menyarung ceremony. Rather, it is a gradual process that ends when the person has become a proficient balien. Similarly, it is expected not that all the balien's symptoms of illness will disappear immediately upon being initiated but that the balien will eventually be cured of his or her illness through the practice of balien cures. The remission of any symptom is attributed to the successful neutralization of spirits. If some other symptoms persist, it is attributed either to spirits who have not yet been captured or to another coexisting pathology.

> One of Bolom's original complaints, constipation, still caused her occasional discomfort over a year after her initiation as a balien. Her husband even bought a book on Malay magic (mujarrobat) in an attempt to find some Islamic charm to cure her. But she felt, and the family agreed, that she had been cured of pais layu-layu inasmuch as she had regained her appetite and ceased having dreams indicative of this illness.

The process of becoming a balien involves an incremental change of attitude, an incorporation of new ways of thinking, and a growing sense of commitment to the role. Besides belief in the efficacy of the initiation as therapy, the cognitive patterns of the balien evolve with practice into a professionalized consciousness.

Notes

1. Dancing is a symptom of the balien's calling, since the baliens dance in their ceremonies.

2. I have found remarkable parallels to dawawa jalu in Candace Slater's study of narratives from Amazonia involving enchanted dolphin-lovers. The following case sounds as if it could have come from one of my Taman informants: "I would be there in the water and, suddenly, I'd want to get out but couldn't. People began approaching me, people who weren't part of my world, wanting to carry me off with them. Often, I ran. . . . It became so I was afraid to go down to the river" (Slater 1994: 176). Slater observes that the narrator senses he has "been singled out for supernatural attention" (Slater 1994: 175). In some of the stories dolphins make their first appearance in dreams. The enchanted dolphin is invisible to all but the object of his or her affection. People experience intense pleasure when they consort with dolphins and are overwhelmed by sadness when the dolphin leaves. "Not infrequently, the man may endure recurring bouts of near madness, running down to the river at all hours, or consuming great heaps of raw fish" (Slater 1994: 185). People visited by dolphins may consult shamans to help them with their plight, but at this point the comparison between the Amazon and the Upper Kapuas ends. The shaman either drives away the dolphin lover by administering baths and fumigations, or instructs the afflicted person or a male family member to kill the dolphin. Although Slater (Slater 1994: 173) refers to dolphin encounters as a culture-bound syndrome, there is no indication that they are perceived as illnesses in and of themselves. And judging from Slater's account, the institution of shamanism is not related to close encounters with dolphins.

3. Besides rice panicles, the following are used to decorate the *sarung ase: suri* (*Cordyline fruticosa*), *banoh* (*Gendarussa vulgaris*), *taraksio* (*Tetractomia obovata*), *Tanpasui* (Zingiberaceae), *tentebong* (*Medinilla* sp.), *riribu* (*Lygodium flexuosum*), *pinang* (*Areca catechu*), *mendor* (unidentified), and *ikan seluang karangas* (a fish, unidentified).

4. This approach to ritual as performance originates in studies by Victor Turner (especially 1968, 1974) and is developed in pertinent ways by Kapferer (1991).

5. The works of Tambiah (1985: 77ff., 123–162) and Atkinson (1989) suggest the necessary function in certain rituals of the presence of an audience merely to be there to receive the actions of performers; paying attention to or understanding the performance may not be as important. Siikala (1978: 61) also stresses the important role of the audience in shamanism.

6. This seems to be the only difference in the cultural elaboration of male and female baliens. The great majority of baliens are women (see Chapter 7). Menyarung is the only Taman ceremony requiring the participation of both male and female baliens. However, King (1985: 192–195) witnessed a memorial ceremony performed by a male and a female balien among the Embaloh, who are culturally close to the Taman.

7. Clothes are changed in the presence of the mixed audience. The Taman are accustomed to changing their clothes without privacy, and traditional norms of modesty are upheld. For example, a woman puts on a fresh skirt before removing the old one she wishes to change out of.

8. This association of the east with the living and the west with the dead figures in balien seances using the *pangait* (Chapter 6) and in concepts of poisons and antidotes (Chapter 3).

9. There is no established text for any of the balien's chants, although there are some standard formulaic flourishes. The balien's expertise and "art of memory" (Yates 1966), if any, derive from an ability to visualize a landscape. Jules-Rosette's (1975: 158) discussion of songs as an "ongoing field of production," improvised within general guidelines and relying on established formulae, seems applicable to balien songs.

10. Percussion music is required in establishing a rhythm for the dance, and it is also important in providing a link to the spirit realm (Needham 1979). It has been pointed out that drumming is conducive to the altered states of consciousness underlying shamanism (Rouget 1980; Neher 1962), but it is interesting to note that drumming is not used in several balien ceremonies in which contact with spirits is required (see Chapter 6).

11. This embodiment of spirits is best explained by what Siikala (1978) calls "ecstatic role-taking," "being" another person by way of identification. Ecstatic role-taking involves the individual's entire being and may take place at different levels of consciousnes.

12. According to one balien, the blossom is stroked three times before it is cracked open. I did not personally notice that.

13. Cash substitutes are made in some cases: Rp 500 for a plate or a knife, Rp 1,000 for a chicken or a ceramic vase. These are very low equivalents. At the end of an all-night mengadengi ceremony, I recorded the following payments: "Payment is given out in the baliens' *taengens* [baskets]. One of the taengens has two bundles of glutinous rice sticks, the others have one each. One person gets a knife and a vase. I think L. gets a cloth but maybe they all do. They [the people holding the ceremony] only have two ceramic bowls, so two baliens are given glass plates instead. Rp 1,000 is given to T. and B., Rp 500 to D., I think in lieu of knives. The other knife goes to L. They get bags of flour [sensagun]. D. and L. get more than seven kilograms of rice, the others get more than three kilograms. L. will get a chicken."

14. When I showed an unusual stone I had found to a woman informant, she asked me whether I had dreamed of it. And when I asked a woman whether the stones elicited in her mengadengi ceremony were connected somehow to her dreams, her reply was (roughly translated), "What do you think?"

15. As King (1975: 108) points out, freshly caught stones are soft, warm, and "putty-like." He also suggests that the balien moulds the stones. Although some stones appear to have been artificially moulded, possibly by carving, I have no evidence that Taman ideology admits this to be the case.

16. A comparison may be made between this piercing and the practice of piercing the penis for the insertion of penis pins (*palang*), which in the past were commonly worn by the Taman and other peoples of Borneo (D. E. Brown 1991, Brown et al. 1988). Like the piercing of the eyes and fingers, the very existence of this practice strains the credulity of those for whom it is not an accepted cultural norm. Donald Brown (personal communication) states that the pins are likened to hooks in native writings on the subject.

17. Luhrmann (1989: 312) has identified this process as "'interpretive drift'— the slow, often unacknowledged shift in someone's manner of interpreting events as they become involved with a particular activity."

6

The Work and
Equipment of the Balien

Having undergone initiation in the menyarung ceremony, the novice balien is empowered to heal patients in the balien's ceremonies. In all, there are seven balien ceremonies, including the menyarung ceremony.[1] These are clearly ranked in complexity and gravity. The balien learns the simpler treatments first and gradually becomes accomplished in the more advanced procedures. The balien's apprehension and use of spirits in these ceremonies require distinctive cognitive modes as well as special equipment and accoutrements. In analyzing the ceremonies in detail, this chapter discusses time outlays, payments, material culture (equipment, accoutrements, and provisions), narrative rhetoric, and discourse.

The Hierarchy of Balien Techniques

Bubut, the first ceremony, comprises the first level of therapy. In it, the balien rubs over the patient's body stones dipped into a crushed medicinal plant, magically extracting the disease as if through magnetism. *Mangait,* the next level, is the location of the patient's lost soul by the balien, who offers a replica of it to the spirits, and instructs the patient's family where the soul has been taken so that another replica can be exchanged for the patient's soul. In this ceremony the balien uses stones that take him or her on a trip via waterways to disused swidden fields, graveyards, fig trees, ditches, or other "haunted" places to find the lost soul. In *malai,* the balien goes to the spot where the patient's soul has been located, snatches it from the spirit that has taken it, and brings it back to the patient, reinserting it into the fontanel of the head. *Menindoani,* the next level, is an advanced variation of mangait, made more difficult by the fact that the balien's soul must "fly" in the air and reach the land of the dead to catch the additional souls that have strayed too far to be caught through mangait. In *tabak buse,* baliens beat drums to communicate with the spirits. In *mengadengi,* spirits causing illness through disturbance are neutralized by being snatched out of the air and turned to stone. The final ceremony, menyarung, continues the process begun in mengadengi in a longer and more elaborate ceremony culminating in the initiation of the person, who is no longer a patient but an inductee. The menyarung ceremony is the pinnacle of the balien system and also its pivot, since it creates a cycle by producing both baliens and the stones they need to perform all healing ceremonies. This cycle is reproductive and perpetuates the balien system (see Figure 6.1).

These seven therapies and ceremonies may be grouped into three categories that are derived from their implicit "ontological assumptions" (Boyer 1993): bubut, for removing a pathogenic object or spirit being from the body; mangait, malai, menindoani, and tabak buse, for locating and restoring an errant soul; and mengadengi and menyarung, for capturing free spirits and neutralizing them by turning them into stone.

Figure 6.1 The Balien Ceremonial System as a Cycle

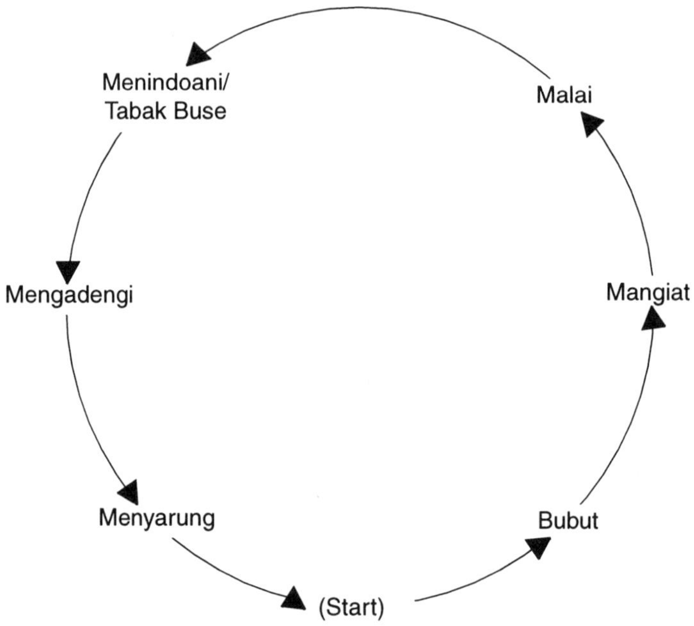

Bubut

Bubut is a therapy in which the balien's stones are stroked over the body to remove spirits or objects sent by spirits. Illnesses that can be treated with this technique are those caused by attacks not to the victim's body but to one of his or her multiple souls. Injuries caused by physical blows to or punctures of the body cannot be cured by bubut. The Malay root word "bubut" means "to pluck or extract," but I am unaware of the existence outside the Upper Kapuas area of the therapeutic procedure described here or of the term "bubut" being used to describe the motion used by the balien in this treatment.

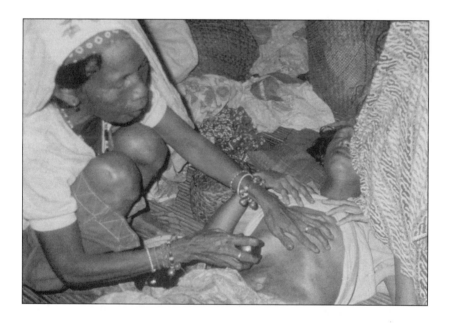

Bubut—disease extraction using stones.

Bubut is the most common and routine form of therapy in the balien's repertoire, yet it is the most significant medically. There is in bubut the physical examination of the patient's body by the knowledgeable hands of the healer, the rubbing of medicinal herbs, a diagnostic interview or conversation in which the history of the complaint is recounted, the removal of a physical object representing the disease object, and the balien's explanation of the disease.

The Use of Stones

The balien's stones are the crucial instruments needed in performing bubut. According to the baliens' ideology, it is the stones that remove the disease-object and cure illness. The stones used must be authentic balien stones (*batu balien*) obtained in the menyarung ceremony, not ordinary stones (batu karangan). I once asked an informant why ordinary stones must not be used, and how he was sure such stones were not in the baliens' baskets. He answered pointedly with a rhetorical question: If they were regular stones, how could they cure anything? Informants stated without exception that baliens' stones are from sai; they were caught in the menyarung ceremony, and they could not possibly be ordinary stones. I have never heard a Taman person even slightly doubt this proposition. Even an informant who did not believe in baliens, and who said the baliens' syndrome was a result of their overactive imaginations, turned very serious when I suggested that their stones were ordinary ones collected in the river.

The balien's obligation to perform bubut on anyone requesting it is imposed by the stones: It is believed that if they are not used to cure people, the balien's original sickness will return. Furthermore, nonbaliens cannot use the stones to cure, since they cannot feel the sai, their fingertips not having been pierced with metal hooks (see Chapter 5). Even a person who has obtained stones through the mengadengi ceremony but has not undergone menyarung cannot cure patients, though the stones produced in that ceremony are potent and authentic balien stones.

A balien first becomes proficient at bubut by practicing on household members. Eventually, someone outside the household will request a bubut. Very likely, the first requests will come from family members in the village, but it is not long before a new balien will get requests from others. Novice baliens are distinctly less proficient in the sleight-of-hand technique involved in bubut than experienced ones, who can skillfully drop even large, heavy pebbles into their bowls without it being apparent that they have been palmed. This technique is mastered over time.

Bubut begins with an invocation of the stones, goading them to remove the disease. The balien covers his or her head with a large cloth, makes an offering of rice to the spirits of the deceased baliens, and while rubbing a stone over the body intones the following:

Ikonamanah sarin,	Heal the patient,
ikonamanah pisin,	cure the patient,
daenau malindung rabe dinten dada dingin.	remove the spirit in the stomach.
Dangkatan arengan kole' a mintuarin.	Make the body light.
Nanasari alayu rabe binten pangolen.	Draw out the stone so that it falls into the bowl.
Bawa' ki' turun tamang manangan batu.	We are embarrassed in front of those who initiated us if this person does not get well.
Ikonna manyoruh alaya jo pais lukaan.	Make the sickness come out.

While performing the bubut the balien will press deep into the flesh to locate the point where the disease entered. A stone that has been dipped in decoctions of crushed herbs—either tantamu or *saur* (*Kaempferia galanga*)—is rubbed slowly over the part of the body. First one stone will be used, then another. Bringing a ceramic bowl near the part of the body being rubbed, the balien produces from under the stone a pebble that makes a sound as it falls into the bowl. The balien massages several parts of the body in this way to rid the patient's body of all disease, squeezing and sometimes blowing on the flesh.

The stones used in the bubut are a sample of a much larger group of stones collected in the initiation ceremony. These stones are kept in a small woven kit (*baranai*) placed at the top of the balien's basket (*taengen*), which contains the rest of the stones as well as other equipment. These stones kept in the baranai include all the tamang, "doubles" of the balien and his or her family members in a mystical sense (see Chapter 5). Besides the tamang, other stones with specialized functions that may be kept in the baranai are Batu Induayo (a female ghost), Batu Antu Anak (a male ghost), *Batu Lidah* ("tongue stone," for removing spirits from the stomach), and a number of stones from animal spirits.

The bubut is classified by the kind of stone used—for example, *bubutan lalawi* (tortoise bubut)—or by the kind of object extracted. In general, the stones of water animals are associated with illnesses of the stomach and digestive tract, and the stones of land animals and birds are associated with illnesses of the head. This may be related to a distinction in the spirit world geography between the river and the forest. There was some variation and discrepancy among both baliens and nonbaliens regarding which kinds of bubut treat which illnesses, suggesting that this knowledge is not highly standardized.

In effect, the nature of the illness is described or specified by the kind of stone used to remove it. Pebbles removed in the bubut are believed to be pathogenic spirits, possibly in the same category as the spirits of the stones used to remove them from the body. The pebbles must be "fed" to the bubut stones so that they do not fly into the balien's body.

Some removed objects also have specific names and guidelines. The most dangerous object removed by the balien is the *tampun,* a long stone removed from the head. A special set of customs pertain to ensure that the disease does not enter the balien's body if a tampun is removed. The tampun must be cut out with a small knife (parang), and the balien must be paid a quantity of glutinous rice, an egg, and a chicken. If the patient does not consent to this payment, a regular bubut may be performed instead. In *bubutan antu anak* (for illnesses affecting the heart), an object looking like a worm is supposedly taken out. Similarly, in *bubutan munusi* (removal of a disease-object from deep within the body), the balien must be paid with particular kinds of objects: a knife, a chicken, and a plate.

The Use of Medicines

The balien performing the bubut cure uses one of two medicines, crushed herbs into which the stones are dipped before they are stroked over the patient's body. Decoctions of either tantamu or saur may be used. Tantamu is considered more appropriate for treating adults, and saur more appropriate for children, but these indications are not adhered to rigidly. The medicines are used to bring the sai to the surface so that it can be caught, much as poison to stupefy fish is used to bring them to the surface of the river. This use of herbs may elucidate King's (1975) description of the balien's stone as acting "something like a magnet, containing a spiritual force that attracts the 'sickness' from the patient's body." Both of the bubut medicines have a pleasant aroma and produce a pleasant sensation when rubbed on the skin.

Tantamu has a pungent, aromatic fragrance and a sharp, bitter flavor. In Indonesian traditional medicine, the herb has some fifty uses for constipation and other stomach ailments, fever, and ailments of the gall bladder and liver. Tantamu stimulates the gall bladder in producing bile and improves circulation in the blood vessels. (The rhizome has a volatile oil content of 8 percent [Dharma 1985: 265–266], containing phellandrene, turmerol, curcumin, calcium, camphor, glycoside, toluol methyl-carbinol, and 1-cycloisoprene myrcene [Tampubolon 1981: 117].) It may have some anaesthetic or analgesic properties, which would explain its use in the piercing ceremonies. Most baliens grow this plant in their gardens, and if they are working at the houses of clients who do not have it on hand, it can usually be borrowed from a neighbor. Desiccated tantamu is often found in baliens' kits, but fresh rhizomes must be cut each time a balien practices. Saur contains borneol, camphor, cineole, and ethyl alcohol (Tampubolon 1981: 71). Its rhizome is popular in Indonesia not only as a tonic but as a spice. Baliens use only the succulent leaves, not the rhizome, medicinally.

Cases

The usual time for these treatments is in the evening, around supper time. Early in the morning is also a common time to make a call, especially if a person has been sick all night. Once the day's work has started, it is often more difficult to find a particular balien. Judging from many informants' statements, it is considered virtually a taboo to call on a balien in the middle of the day, when the sun is hot. Explanations such as "The medicine won't take" are offered. Despite this, baliens are sometimes called on in midday because "if you are in great pain you cannot stand to wait."

As far as I can determine, baliens are always willing to treat all prospective patients unless they are unavailable due to their own illness or simply not at home. The popularity of certain baliens explains why inexperienced ones are called into service: The preferred balien is not available when needed. Frequently, a sick person will be bubut-ed by several baliens sequentially. Convenience seems to be the main criterion in selecting a balien for bubut service.

A family or group of single people come together to the home of a balien. Each person wanting to be treated brings a cup of rice in payment. The balien asks what the sickness is, then brings the patient into the inner part of the house where the stones are kept. The conversation is a mixture of talk about everyday concerns and the nature of the illness and its possible origin. The balien may ask questions to learn how the illness started and how long it has lasted. The balien also palpates the patient's body and examines visible symptoms.

The following case exemplifies the clinical evaluation of illness that occurs in the setting of the bubut.

> Case 1: *Bubutan sai* [spirit bubut]. Two women come in, one bringing a covered cup filled with rice and the other holding a two- or three-year-old girl. The mother said the child was hot, had been sick for "a long time," and cried all night. She said they had to find a balien and that the baby had to be cured through bubut. The more the girl cried, the sicker she got, the mother said. The girl was whimpering, and her throat was swollen (*bambang*). The balien stroked her stones on the child's forehead. The balien, trying to diagnose the disease while bubut-ing the baby, said that if it were fire badi, the color [inside the throat] would be as red as a red skirt, accompanied by swelling. She observed that there was no redness. Continuing her bubut cure, she asked whether the family had put up a fence. She was considering the possibility that the sickness was caused by stake badi. She went back to something the patient's mother had previously mentioned. "Was the child already treated by mangait therapy by Mina [another balien]? Why didn't you say so?" The mother then admitted that there was a fence at their swidden field hut. The balien explained that the fence in question is not hers but her parents'. But the woman protested the line of reasoning the balien was taking, noting that her father never makes fences. With this information, the balien makes a diagnosis of "internal cut," dasumpit jalu ["shot by a spirit being"], which she removes. But she observes that the area is about to become a boil, and advises the mother to take the child to Putussibau for an injection. "Someone is going downstream. Try to go along." After the bubut, the balien throws a few grains of rice on her stones and drops a few through the floor slats.

From this case it is evident that the balien obtained a significant amount of information from physical (usually deep) palpation and the close-up inspection that goes along with it. Following up on a hunch, the balien asked questions. Through dialogue, she constructed a medical case history and attempted to elicit information to fit the presenting symptoms and complaints with an interpretation of spirit revenge.

> Case 2: *Bubutan jalu lawai (duduri).* A thirteen-year-old girl from another part of the village is brought in by her mother at 7:30 a.m. She has a stomach ache. She is first given a head bubut, then a stomach bubut. The stomach is pressed in. Now that the child has been treated, the mother is given

a head bubut; she complains that her vision is "dark" [*araun mata'an*]. Now the mother's stomach is also bubut-ed, first lower then upper abdomen, which she says is painful. Her lower rib area is rubbed by the balien. After being treated they both sit in the front room again.

In this case a child is brought by her mother because of a stomachache, but the balien medicates not only her stomach but her head. Following this treatment her mother, who had accompanied the girl, receives the same treatment.

The bubut ceremony epitomizes the importance of stones as apparatuses of the balien's profession, capable of locating and extracting spirits and disease-objects. The use of stones in this ceremony functions to create a nonverbal medical discourse in which the etiology and meaning of the disease are specified in terms of spirit attack. Taman concepts of physiology and pathology are exemplified in this removal by healing specialists of disease entities with these stones that are themselves from spirits. Finally, the bubut is an arena for a clinical assessment of symptoms and the construction of a medical case history.

Mangait

Mangait is the first of the balien's seance ceremonies, which are part of the second level of the balien's work. The seance technique, using the pangait, is continued at a more advanced level in the menindoani and tabak buse ceremonies. In performing these seances, baliens use what Harner (1980: 59ff.) calls the "shamanic state of consciousness," which is different from the state of awareness employed in the bubut technique.

The name of the mangait ceremony is derived from the root word "kait," meaning "hook" or "hook figure." This etymology is also the origin of the term for the main piece of equipment used in this ceremony, the pangait, a smooth wooden pole fitted with a hook-shaped metal tip. This pole enables the balien to harness the power of stones and contact the spirit world by taking the balien's soul out of the body and on a trip. The pangait is thought of as a ladder or staircase leading to the spirit world.[2] Through the vehicle of the pangait, the balien speaks to the stones, directing them to take the balien where he or she wants to go. The pangait enables the balien not only to speak to but to hear the stones. It also allows the balien to see both the spirits and the soul of the patient and thus to know more about the nature of the illness than is possible with the bubut alone. It is by using the pangait, therefore, that the balien functions as a shaman—using soul travel to heal a sick person.

As discussed in Chapter 5, the hook motif is a complex symbol providing a center of gravity to the balien's work. It replicates and reiterates the emblematic symbolism of the rabe (the hook inserted in the eyes and fingertips of the initiate) and the tips of the areca blossom cracked open in the menyarung ceremony. But in the former its meaning for the balien appears to derive from its use in the mangait. As Harrisson observes (1965: 342), "The fish hook represents the bringing down, the hooking on, up above, of the spirit elements."

This ceremony requires the use of all the balien's stones in the balien's carrying basket, not only those used in the bubut.[3] While bubut stones are polished and have individual and often humanized identities, the rest of the stones, called batu kait because of their association with the pangait and the mangait ceremony, are associated with animals or unknown spirits and lack individualized identities or names. Batu kait are crude, rough, and usually larger than bubut stones, and they carry the balien's soul.

Selection of a Balien

To serve in a mangait service, a balien must be contracted for the whole night. Around twilight, a child or other family member is enlisted to call on the chosen balien. If the balien is available, the stones and the pangait are taken back to the house of the sick person. If the balien is unavailable, another balien will be sought if the messenger has been authorized to do so.

Since this therapy lasts the entire evening, it is not possible for a balien to perform mangait in more than one household in a night. Furthermore, according to custom, the stones may not leave the house after nightfall. A few baliens are in the greatest demand for the mangait service, and they must often decline requests to serve because of a prior engagement. As the son of a popular balien explained to the prospective client, "Mother's stones have already been taken." Even though the cost of the mangait service is small, some weight is attached to the decision of whom to call. Baliens are sometimes called from adjacent villages, and more than occasionally from their swidden field residences (*langko uma*). A balien who travels a significant distance must be escorted home, probably the following morning. This extra time and effort adds to the true cost of the ceremony. A strong correlation exists between the longhouse or village unit (banua) of the client and the favored balien; this appears to be based more on kinship and association than on physical proximity. Clients may travel long distances to call on baliens who are family members.

Case 3: A balien, Kasien, had been called from Nibung, a swidden field area several kilometers upstream from the village of Sibau Hilir, to heal a woman who was suffering from stomach pains and could not get out of bed. Her husband, who had brought Kasien to the village, said at first that he asked for her help because she was *sarasian* [fitting, matching]. She is his father's younger sister. He had tried another balien who performed a kind of bubut called bubutan munusi, but the illness had returned after getting better temporarily. He didn't call a male balien who lives permanently in Nibung because he was elsewhere, at a party celebrating the end of prohibitions following a funeral. That man would also have been a good choice. After I interviewed him about several other baliens, the man admitted that the most *rasi* [compatible, harmonious] balien would be another balien, Tanduk, but that she had already been contracted by her own son, and that he was not sure whether Kasien was sarasian.

Equipment and Materials

Before mangait is performed, the pangait is set up pointing eastward—the direction of the rising sun—and is tied with a cloth to a house post. The bottom of the pole is grounded in or beside the basket containing the balien's stones.

The first time a novice balien performs mangait, she or he borrows another balien's pangait. In payment, a hook tip is forged and fashioned by the client and given to the balien in payment (see Figure 6.2). The tip is then fitted and attached with twine to a hardwood pole made of *balawan* wood (*Tristania*) about six feet long, smoothed and blackened with clay. The instrument is usually stored by the hearth.

An essential accoutrement used in this ceremony is the *tauning*, bracelets of colored beads and cast-iron bells. Before beginning any treatment, the balien must have the bracelets tied on. (When baliens work coop-

Figure 6.2 Pangait Tip (tracing, reduced to 65 percent)

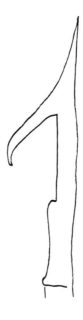

eratively they tie on each other's bracelets.) Each balien possesses two tauning. They make a jingling sound when the balien shakes her wrists or pulls down on the pangait in this ceremony, and this is thought to attract the spirits.

Two small statues known as *sulekale* are prepared for the mangait ceremony, usually by a man in the patient's household. These are pieces of sugar cane about 2 inches long, carved roughly into the shape of a person and wrapped with pieces of cloth in the form of a skirt if the patient is a female and in the form of a breechcloth if the patient is a male. These statues are put on top of a cup of uncooked glutinous rice (*pulut*), which itself sits on top of a bowl of uncooked regular rice. The statues are later offered to the spirits in exchange for the patient's soul.

Finally, the balien needs a cloth (*kain burih*) for covering the upper body while performing the ceremony. According to custom, a cloth with a printed pattern is provided as a gift the first time mangait is performed, but it is not certain that the balien must use this cloth in subsequent mangait ceremonies.

Altered State of Awareness

During mangait ceremonies the balien seems to be in a semi–trance state, dissociated from the material and human world. By enclosing themselves with their stones under a cloth or blanket, baliens facilitate communion with spirit familiars and soul travel enabling contact with other spirits. This act of covering also serves to separate the balien from the mundane world (cf. Gell 1980). The use of polek mo (a magical oil rubbed on the balien's face and hands and on the pangait) and the cutting of the outer tissue of the eye believed to take place during the menyarung ceremony, enable the balien to see spirits that are invisible to ordinary people. Baliens claim they can see the spirits as light or hear their voices while performing mangait, though they cannot make lucid statements about the nature of their encounters and cannot even remember them well. One balien I interviewed said: "In mangait we don't see. The stones take us traveling to the place where the sick person's soul is, and tell us [where it is]. It's like a dream. The stone says, 'over there.' The soul travels."

From the balien's point of view, mangait is a far greater challenge than bubut because the encounter with sai is considered frightening. The fact that several baliens are incapable of performing mangait can be explained by this fear.

> Rea reassured Samarai [a woman who was being treated by baliens and was herself being groomed as a candidate balien], "it is up to you if you don't want to perform mangait." (Previously, Samarai had said that she was afraid of spirits, afraid to perform mangait, and that if required to catch the soul in malai, the other baliens would have to go ahead of her, that is, to lead her.) Rea said she was taught not by two or three people, but just one.

At first she was also frightened. She said that if her teacher took them, they (their souls) would travel as far as Sanalan lake in Eko Tambai village. In menindoani, they would get as far as a very long longhouse, a place where the ghosts play, until they met the souls of young girls, making *songket* cloth. Rea would go along with her, just learning. In the future, when she becomes knowledgeable, then she can lead (teach), and her junior colleagues will come along.

As can be seen in the following case, the balien's chant in mangait not only narrates but also directs the flight of her soul to the various places where the culprit spirit has taken the patient's soul. The balien is aided by spirit helpers, the named tamang stones. The chant describes things seen (bathing children) and activities occurring in not the material plane but the spirit plane. She also sees what the spirit is doing to the sick girl's soul (spearing it like a pig) and commands it to stop. In return for the girl's soul, she offers the statue. Then she directs the way back home, stopping first at a graveyard and cautioning the stones who are steering the speedboat to avoid driftwood.

Soul Travel

Case 4: In treating a ten-year-old girl, a balien talks directly to the stones in the everyday Taman language. She first recites an incantation (*sampi*) to the statue:

Sulekale, take the soul,
substitute for the soul that has your face.
Probably there is someone [a spirit] who is attracted to you
You are desired by him.
Wherever I follow,
I take this to replace your body.
I take a spirit (*pemari'an*) to the rear of the house or the front of the house.
I take it to the place for entertaining guests [the front of the house].
Return to the stone building.
I bring this substitute for your body to the field or to wherever you are.
Come home safely, carefully.
I bring it to the graveyard, to replace your body so health returns, like normal, beautiful like the body of a youth, a maiden, body of D., body of K., body of A.,[4] come home together as a family!
Safely.
Sundar, Grandmother Tutumanen [names of female stones].
Male balien stones, Selorgai, Tuladang Pongan, Bunut Turing, Lalayang Bajubu', Tinang Baro.

Let's go!
One, two, three, four, five, six, seven!

The balien is almost ready to begin the mangait ceremony. She says, "I just want to drink a little," drinks from a cup of *marem* (palm wine) prepared for her, and bites the blade of her sword (a ceremonial action intended to strengthen her soul), then places it under her right foot. This action, called *pangaran batak ngano,* is also intended to strengthen the soul. She crouches over the suspended stick and her stones, covers her entire body and basket containing her stones with a cloth or blanket, and begins her chant.[5]

The opening recitation is directed in part to the statue, in part to the errant soul of the sick person and the souls of the family members, and finally to the stones that will help her on her journey, which she addresses by name:

> Drink up! We're leaving. Reach Siang [the patient], find her together, as a family.
> Whoo! Let's go! Bunut Turing Menungan [name of stone]. Pinang Andan [the leading stone, the oldest].
> Finished smoking, chew betel.
> Ehh! Lead the way, Bunut Turing, Tingang Barang, Lalayang Bajubo' . . .
> Embark! Travel! Come home, you bathing children are ordered home.
> We are going straight to the field.
> Ooh! Ooooh! Isen ["beloved" or "brother"],[6] we are entering to take the soul, disease don't play games with my grandchild![7]

> The disused rice field. Where's the place? Not here. Look around . . . very carefully. . . . We meet in the river. Siang, don't let 'em lie to you like that, he's messing around, she'll be hurt with a knife. Don't let him treat you like that, she'll be shot by a blowdart. She's not a boar, not an animal. Here's a statue to substitute for her.

> Take this and beat it as a substitute for her body. This child, don't beat her like that. (Pull out this wood.) [Said to the soul of the sick child.]

> You can't do that. For what is she being speared, she's done no harm. You can't treat a child like that, this is why she has a backache, a stomach ache. Your house will be attacked.

> Come home, all of you come home! [Said to the patient's soul as the balien pulls down on the pangait, rattling the bells in her bracelets.]

> Don't be attached to the child of this person, she is without fault.

> Together as brothers and sisters, don't harm this human child.
> Come home, all of you come home [said to the stones].
> Come home using the same path as the first one.
> Stay a second at the house [swidden field hut].
> Go across the river to the graveyard.
> No one's here.
> How can we go home, where's the boat?
> Careful steering the motor.
> Careful or we'll hit driftwood.
> Here we are [at the graveyard].

They say no one's home.
Open the door.
Hopefully no one's been hidden away here.
Come on, let's go home.
Careful, we're using the speedboat.
Come home, children [pulls down on the pangait].

Following the mangait service, the balien emerges from under the cloth, usually perspiring and in a daze. She is given another drink of palm wine and informs the patient's family where the soul has been taken. In most of the cases I observed, the balien found that the soul had been at the spot of a disused rice field, where it had been taken hostage by a spirit who had been hurt by a stake in the ground. Once, however, a balien had a great air of satisfaction at having found a simple solution to the problem: She told the family that the patient's soul had not been taken by a sai; rather, it was in a small river out behind the house.

At the end of the mangait the balien throws one of the sugarcane sculptures out of the back of the house, offering it to the spirit with words such as the following:

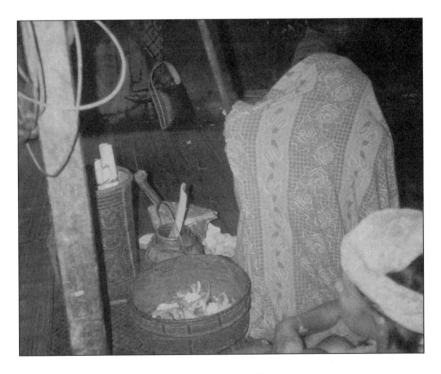

Mangait (seance).

Ninna ipapaisin ingkin.	Take this and hurt it.
Ipuling -ulingan ingkin ito' toi ingkin yang kehendaki ingkin.	This is for your pleasure; this is what you want.
Kutiang pala molek tiang panyule'.	This I take in exchange for the sick person.
Ingkinna loang tambaruang.	Induayo (spirits) conferring in the ground.
Ingkinna antu bua' an.	Ghost in the fruit tree.
Antu kawangan.	Ghost of the *tengkawang* (dipterocarp) tree.
Ninna natikan ipulung -ulungan ingkin.	It is the sulekale that must play with you ghosts.
Ulun pangkawan ulun suruhanan.	As your slave.
Kutiang pala molek doisanon, nanna isanti	This child, she must return together with her mother.
Sialo ingkinna, Siala!	Take this, all of you!
Salo' an nanna sukat barasa.	The sulekale together with cigarettes and rice.
Ipole' ingkin malaman pole damairin.	Return in the middle of the night.

Then, touching the patient, the balien recites a blessing: "*Molek kualakin. Molek isadigin -sadingau. Molek kuponangkin kusule' nana kaletu anak binge.*" ("Come home. I have exchanged a figurine shaped in the form of a maiden for you.")

The following day a member of the family must discard the second figurine in the spot determined by the balien. Depending on the nature of the sickness, the balien may bubut the patient at this point.

Besides the household members of the patient, who arrange for the mangait ceremony, a number of visitors are usually present during this service, usually from the village unit or longhouse in which the ceremony is being held. Many of the visitors are present to receive bubut after or in some cases before the main ceremony. These treatments are not paid for, and the discussion of the complaint is much greatly reduced and simplified compared with those times when a person calls on a balien at the balien's own house. The balien accepts all requests for bubut.

The Neglected Patient

In contrast to the hands-on nature of the balien-patient encounter in bubut, the attention of the balien while performing mangait is directed at the stones or the spirits, or the patient's detached soul that has been taken somewhere else. Meanwhile, the patient in the house is left alone, reclining or being comforted by a family member in another part of the room. The balien works and communicates more with the patient's family members (the group of supporters called "the diagnostic set" by Payne [1985: 337]) than with the patient. Remarkably, the patient, for whom the ceremony is being held, appears at times to be neglected.

Case 5: An eight-year-old boy has been in the hospital for eight to ten days, but showed no sign of improvement, so his grandfather (the village head-man) brought him home. He has dysentery and doesn't want to eat or drink. Food was offered him and he refused all. He also moaned in pain a few times. The house was very full—maybe forty people or more were inside. People came in, touching the boy. Most of the people from the longhouse were there. The balien finished her mangait and said the soul was to be found at the spot of a wooden post in a swidden field located across the river. Then she bubut-ed another woman and paid no attention to the boy in pain. She came back and tapped the patient and another boy on the head. The boy appeared to me to be incredibly sick and thin. But the balien showed no feelings of pity toward him.[8]

Malai

Malai is an extension of mangait, in which the balien, in addition to locat-ing the patient's soul, retrieves and returns the errant soul by taking it out of the clutches of a spirit, bringing it home, and reinserting it into the patient's body. The balien must physically interact with spirits in the phenomenal world. Besides using a pangait and stones, the balien offers food to entice the spirit that is holding the soul. The balien's ointment, polek mo, is used so that the balien can see spirits while remaining invisible to them. From the balien's point of view, malai involves a considerable amount of work. It is also a chance to learn through apprenticeship: being taken along (*ikiring*) is the way for a balien to advance through the ranks of professional accom-plishment.

Among the Sibau Taman but not the Kapuas Taman this ceremony requires the labor of two baliens, a leader and a deputy. Because of the rel-atively steep expense entailed, resources must be accumulated beforehand, and the service may be planned as long as a week in advance. However, in emergencies, an impromptu version of malai, called *maniang aso,* can be performed during the daytime.[9]

The balien's equipment for this ceremony includes several items of tra-ditional women's clothing, including objects no longer part of contemporary Taman apparel: *karimut* (a girdle made from ringlets of silver threaded on rattan), *ganding* (shell bracelets), *telang manik* (a beaded necklace), a bead-ed blouse, and *ampan manik* (a beaded headcloth). In addition, the baliens use their swords (parang), *wase* (a metal object resembling an awl that is struck against the sword), pangait, and their baskets containing stones.[10]

A large woven container (called a *bakol,* according to Harrisson [1965: 260]) holds all the rice being offered. An assistant measures the rice into a smaller basket containing the paraphernalia being used by the baliens. This person (who is not a balien) removes the old rice at each stage of the service, pouring it into a third basket, replacing it with rice from the first basket, and topping it with the baliens' offerings. The rice ends up in a final container from which it is distributed to the baliens in payment for their services.

Preliminaries

The night before malai begins, people gather in the house to stand vigil as the *kangkuang* (a wooden slit gong) is periodically rapped. The family holding this ceremony must provide hospitality for guests, many of whom will spend the night. It is largely the youth who are attracted to such events, where they can play card games or dominoes, while listening to recordings of Malaysian pop music.

The ceremony itself begins the following morning, after the baliens have prepared their equipment. The first part of the ceremony consists of an invitation to the spirits of the great deceased baliens (*balien jolo*), a request to confer with them and offer counsel. A chicken is placed in a bamboo cage at which one of the baliens tosses rice mixed with tantamu while inviting the spirits of the balien jolo to attend. As this is being done, the second, deputized balien strikes the wase with a sword.

The spirits of the baliens who "led us before" are called. Female baliens are called first, then male baliens. The balien jolo are implored to view the illness and send a message through the body of the chicken about its nature and cause, the identity of the spirit causing it, and the cure.

Ketika: *Chicken Oracle*

The chicken trapped in the cage in front of the baliens making their offering is then slaughtered by one of the men. The blood is collected in a bowl and examined with a feather by the leading baliens for signs of the disease from color, irregularities, and texture, especially the existence of bubbles. Next, the stomach and intestines of the chicken are examined, specifically any nodules, for color. If a spirit has inflicted an internal cut (*anggunguran*) in the patient's body, evidence of this can be seen in the blood. Nonbaliens may kibitz over the bowl of blood with the baliens and gave their readings. For example, one woman said that she knew what the illness was, because when her daughter was sick, there were the same patterns in the blood. Some people suggested that *ketika* was a rational system whose meanings are known to the baliens. However, an experienced balien said: "If there is a hole, the baliens, if they are in the situation of malai, can see it in the chicken's blood. If they are just sitting around like we are here, how can they know?" The implication was that the state of consciousness specific to the balien while performing this ceremony permits the balien to commune with spirits and to see things not perceptible through ordinary vision. The balien in malai is receptive to the words of the balien jolo, who provide information about the illness.

> Case 6: In the blood *ketika* (oracle), the baliens say the blood is not yet cleaned, and that there is still some excrement in it. They consider the stomach and note that it is not red, saying that that is good. If it were red it would mean that the person could not get better. The presiding balien says there is an object that "went home" in the form of a stone (evidenced in the knotted intestine). The sick girl received the stone previously when she was sick. The stone was given by a spirit, Grandmother Tutumanen. This is a good sign, but because of it the chicken's intestine is a bit knotted. The baliens can tell its origin from the chicken's stomach.

In another case, a fence in the ground, causing badi, was ascertained by the fact that the blood was black, spotted, and had lumps in it.

Locating, Capturing, and Replacing the Patient's Soul

The baliens rub the vase, pangait, knife, basket, and awl with tantamu and rice. They also rub the magical oil from their bottles onto their bodies and faces to help them see the spirits. Then they perform the mangait ceremony together under a single cloth, using only one pole. This procedure is called *manidu'*. They each drape coverings over their heads, then put a larger overall covering on top. Both baliens' baskets of stones are used, and the pangait is placed between them. Following this service, the baliens then must explain to the audience where they have located the soul. In one instance the patient and her family could not understand the place the baliens were talking about.

> Case 7: The family asked if they had to go to a particular spot. The balien said, not there, but upstream. The patient says, "We've already built a hut there." The balien replies, "Go and look, probably there is a broken pole, wood from nine years ago, already rotten." The patient's brother-in-law says he does not know where the hut is. The spot is the wood in the ground, the balien tries to explain. The patient says they have built a fence around their field hut. The patient's husband says, "the hut on that land is not ours, it's someone else's." The balien says, "Not that, that one is old, but one that is in land not easy to see, in the water."

Through such a process, in which the balien's vision is reconciled with the patient's family's knowledge of the local geography, the patient's soul is located.

After determining both the nature of the illness and the location of the patient's soul, the baliens prepare offerings to be brought to the spot where the soul is. The offerings include rice, chicken parts, woven leaf cubes containing rice, tapered bamboo tubes holding water, and betel quids. The chicken blood used in the ketika is cooked and added to the offerings, which are placed in cracked ceramic bowls. In addition, large leaves are prepared containing the figures of animals drawn in a pasty dough used to make certain cakes. Two sugarcane figurines (sulekale) are placed in the large leaf offering and one each in the smaller leaf offerings.

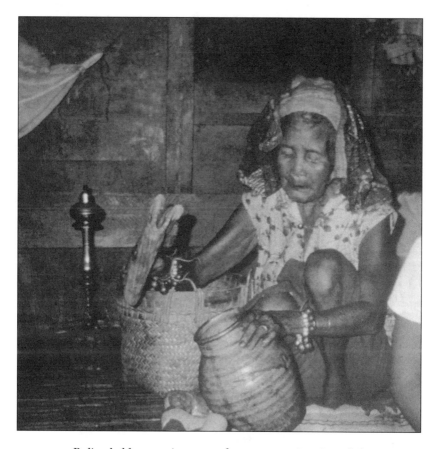

Balien holds ceramic vase and woven container in malai.

After a recess for lunch, the leading balien waves a basket containing the offerings behind the patient's back while the assisting balien strikes the awl against the sword. Then the whole family and as many people in the audience as possible grab with one hand the large basket containing the food offerings.

A small party of the patient's supporters depart either on foot or by boat to the spot where the soul must be caught. Here is a description of one such occasion:

Case 8: Many people accompany the two baliens on a long walk to the spot where they will catch the soul. We have to cross log bridges to get there. The baliens put magical oil on themselves to help them see the spirits after setting up a place by a felled tree at the rice field. They put one big cloth covering both of them over their heads. They sit, placing their swords under their feet. The offering has been hung on the tree stump. They chant briefly. The leading balien runs to catch something, and her deputy grabs a rice plant; these are put in a covered cup. The baliens have caught the soul of the patient. We depart. Outside the field we stop to eat the rice sticks and chicken. Then everyone screams "Wooh!" and we go home as one man strikes the awl and another strikes the vase during the entire procession homeward.

Baliens, and those accompanying them, must partake of the food that has been offered to the spirits in order to prevent anyone from suffering the consequences of kempunan (see Chapter 4). In addition to the other offerings, the figurine is given as a token of exchange for the patient's soul.

The baliens use the same equipment and procedure in malai that are used in the seance technique used in mangait. But the purpose of malai is the opposite of a seance: Rather than drawing the balien's soul outside his or her own body and into the plane of spirits, malai is supposed to invoke or summon the spirits that are in the vicinity, making them and any human souls they are holding visible to and palpable by the baliens, enabling the baliens to snatch them away from the spirits' grip. This conjuring technique is similar to that used in catching stones in the menyarung ceremony.

Upon returning home with the patient's soul, one of the baliens covers herself and the patient's head with a cloth, supposedly putting the small stone into the patient's fontanel, thus replacing an errant soul. (As with the piercing of the candidate balien in the menyarung ceremony, this part of the ceremony is hidden from the view of the spectators.) Bubut-ing of the rest of the patient's body continues, and when this is finished, anyone else requesting a bubut is served.

Menindoani

Menindoani is an extension of malai, beginning at night and lasting several hours. I personally observed it only twice, and in a village it will be performed only a few times a year. The occasions in which menindoani is performed can clearly be divided into those that are planned well in advance and those that are hastily arranged in emergencies. Menindoani is performed only when the patient's soul is considered to be in grave jeopardy. The expense for this service (including the malai held earlier in the day) is rather steep, estimated as the equivalent of about Rp 35,000, more than an average family typically has on hand at a given time. For these ceremonies cooperation is expected from extended family members, and guests sometimes make small prestations of rice.

One of the two cases of menindoani I observed involved the ongoing sicknesses of a mother and her adult daughter as well as a significant dream: Someone saw the younger woman in a dream with a deceased person. In this instance the family was able to plan the ceremony more than a week in advance. In the other case I observed, the woman for whom the ceremony was being held had been sick for some months and was rapidly becoming sicker. Her family became gravely concerned and called a balien to perform mangait, in which it was determined that her soul had drifted far and needed menindoani treatment, and a *kombong* (balien meeting) was held at which plans were made. She underwent malai and menindoani from an established balien assisted by a novice. A few days afterward, she died.

Like mangait and malai, menindoani uses a seance technique involving soul travel. But while the former ceremonies involve travel on earthly terrain only, menindoani requires a further step, to heavenly flight. Among the miraculous stories about the work of the balien, it is said that a balien whose soul is in flight can name the towns and cities she is passing in their correct order even though she has neither traveled far nor been educated. Furthermore, baliens are attributed with an ability to see if someone will soon die, or if a person who has been on a long trip will soon return. The balien's soul travels as far away as Sarawak, Pontianak, or Jakarta during these trips. The menindoani ceremony epitomizes Eliade's (1964: 5) characterization of the shaman's technique as involving soul travel to a non-earthly realm, be it an upper world or a lower world. (No balien technique involves travel to a spirit underworld, as far as I know.)

Menindoani needs to be understood not simply under the rubrics of curing and medicine but also in terms of Taman notions of the perils of the soul. This is evident in the fact that the ceremony may be scheduled in reaction to inauspicious dreams and deaths in the family, to sever relations between the dead and the living. Two baliens I interviewed said, "In malai we catch one soul and put it back in the head. Menindoani is carried out that night to call back any additional souls that may still be missing." Menindoani is the cure for illness and other danger caused by contact with ghosts of dead people. One informant said, "Menindoani is for sickness from dead people; the soul has been taken by a dead person." This statement explains the performance of menindoani in cases of the death of a relative or a dream of a living person being with a dead person. Menindoani is sometimes performed to separate the dead from the living. I was told that the ceremony should be performed a few months after a death so that "the souls of the dead don't mix with the living," causing illness.

Menindoani may be performed by either one or two baliens. In one case I studied, a novice initiated less than a year previously participated. The senior balien led the chant and the junior one followed her every word, repeating it in a low voice. The chance to work in this way is considered a useful opportunity to advance one's standing as a balien, and junior baliens travel with senior baliens to other villages in order to learn the technique.

The client is required to provide a cloth called kain burih as a gift to the spirits when contracting this ceremony. Added to the other offerings in the basket is a bundle of sixty twigs of *tabas pusa'* (*Clerodendrum* cf. *squamatum*) known as *bala buloh,* an offering to Grandmother Siunsun Amas, the "ancestress" of the baliens.

The technique of soul flight in menindoani necessitates the use of a distinct chant, *timang manik* (rising-up chant), and a specific stone, Batu Bau (eagle stone)—one of the many crude stones, batu kait, in the balien's basket—to carry the balien's soul to heaven. During the occasions observed, the chant ran from one to two hours.

The balien's soul eventually reaches Yang Suka and the house of the dead souls. It is believed that the soul has wandered and has been tempted to stay in heaven. On reaching the soul of the patient, the balien can see that person's face inside a ceramic jar. As in mangait, the person's soul is coached home. The following excerpts denote contact with the land of the dead and indicate in a disjointed way the balien's preternatural visions during the ceremony.

> Here we have reached the grave.
> Baliens who are at the grave.
> Carefully see the soul.
> Look in each cape.
> Probably there is a soul lost at the shoreline.
> Look through the corners of broken wood in the place of the dead people.
> Look at the *banang* wood held by ghosts.
> Don't let the soul take shelter there.
> The headdress is dried out at the corner of the pathway of ghosts
> Not yet old, the one with signs of broken wood is still young.
> Come home. Don't you know the previous route?
> People who died as young men and women, there's the place.
> There is the place of the people who have died.
> How do we know? We are just following.
> Search together at the edge of the water.
> Take turns.
> Probably there is an ailing soul [lost on the path].
> Village of ghosts.
> All the villages have been passed.
> Jump to the top. No energy to climb [Mount Tilung].

> [The souls are] eating *embang* fruit.
> Alas, naked children. I am afraid to look at the child. What is being done like this?
> I don't see a child who is still alive.
> Come home! Bate'! [a bridge, the sides of which have been planted with sharpened bamboo].
> I can't see the ghosts. The sick person is covered with leaves, take them off and see.
> You may not see.
> Waters of Jamalu' River.
> Fruit split open by a ghost.
> The soul of the sick person has covered herself with leaves.

The balien's trip in the menindoani ceremony is considered especially dangerous because of the unwholesomeness of contact with dead souls. As mentioned in Chapter 4, acceptance in the house of dead souls is considered a sign of impending death. In one chant, a balien described seeing naked people—the souls of the recently dead, just arrived in heaven—and being frightened by them. The souls encountered say that they do not want to return to the land of the living and that they practically want to remain with the spirits of the dead. Another obstacle on the trip is the bridges and rivers that are passable to the dead but change their size when a living person tries to cross them.

Tabak Buse

This service is very rarely performed (about once a year, at most) and is similar in purpose and elevation to menindoani. My informants have rarely witnessed it, and it appears to be dying out among the Taman. (Several people told me that tabak buse was not a healing ceremony at all but a celebration or thanksgiving.) As far as I know, the ceremony was conducted only once in a Taman village during the entire period of my research. (Unfortunately, I was not present at the time.) Several members of a family had been ill for a long time, and one, an emaciated and apparently tubercular adolescent boy, was a subject of particular concern. The entire family was treated together in the tabak buse ceremony. Two baliens performed the ceremony, a junior (though highly regarded) balien and a more senior balien from an adjacent village.

Baliens use the same chant (timang manik) in performing tabak buse as in menindoani, but in other respects use a completely different procedure, beating a drum for two consecutive nights. (The term "tabak buse" literally refers to the beating of the drum.) Some informants said that while menindoani is used in cases of disease from within the vicinity, in tabak buse the balien's soul travels "straight to heaven" to find the source of the illness. Some Taman said that tabak buse was more expensive to hold than menindoani; the total cost was estimated to be Rp 30,000–40,000.

Harrisson (1965: 262–263) seems to describe what my informants called tabak buse in his account of a ceremony called Belian Maniang Buluh Ayu Sera. He also describes another ceremony I did not observe or hear about, Belian Maniang Ra Buluh Ayu Dua, in which two buluh ayu (decorated bamboo) poles are employed, and the quantities of rice and glutinous rice required are doubled. (*Dua* means "two" and *sera* means "one.")

Mengadengi

Mengadengi is the capture of stones in a nightlong ceremony, the purpose of which is to neutralize spirits disturbing the victim of pais layu-layu. The word "mengadengi" is an elaboration of the Taman root *kadeng,* which means "to stand"; "mengadengi" means "to stand (someone) up." Informants deny that this etymology is pertinent, but based on this etymology "mengadengi" can be said to be the opposite of "menindoani," which derives from *tindo'an,* meaning "bed" or "longhouse apartment" (*tindo'* means "sleep"). So according to the rules of grammar, "menindoani" should mean "to bring home," or "to put to bed," and by extension, "to lay (someone) down." The reason for this opposition (an opposition by no means present in the awareness of Taman informants) is unclear; however, menindoani marks the end of one phase of therapy—the treatment of illnesses caused by spirit attack, effected by the return of errant or captured souls. By contrast, mengadengi is the beginning of another process, one that culminates in a person's becoming a balien. Menindoani, like mangait before it, conducts the balien's soul to the place of spirits, but in mengadengi, the balien's soul does not travel. As in the second part of malai, the pangait and stones are used here to broadcast the balien's voice to the spirits but with the opposite purpose: to conjure them, that is, to attract them to the site of the ceremony.

Some similarities between mengadengi and menindoani should be noted. Either ceremony may be performed in treating cases of illness associated with pais layu-layu. The decision to perform mengadengi rather than menindoani is based on subtle differences in the characteristics of the patient's illness and other factors. Menindoani could be followed by the recommendation that a person should also undergo mengadengi. In any case, the recipient of mengadengi must first be treated with malai earlier in the day. Like menindoani, mengadengi is a complex ceremony performed at night that takes several hours to complete.

Unlike menindoani or any of the other previous therapies, the patient may participate in the therapy by dancing if he or she wishes. Those who have accepted their fate and expect to become baliens dance and converse with the baliens. In other cases, especially when a person is being treated reluctantly, at the insistence of family members, the patient may sit nearby. A patient may also be too infirm or too young to take part in dancing.

In form, the mengadengi ceremony is a scaled-down version of the menyarung ceremony, in which wild spirits are petrified. Fewer and less elaborate offerings are required in mengadengi than in menyarung, and these may be held in a raised metal tray (*par*) rather than a kalangkang. The kalangkang may also be borrowed from a neighbor, though it must be decorated with fresh leaves and flowers. In contrast with menyarung, which is a planned event, the need to hold mengadengi is generally viewed as being akin to a medical emergency. With this pressing need in mind, baliens may proceed with the ceremony even though not all the required offerings have been assembled. As few as two baliens may participate, though a larger number is preferable. At the conclusion of mengadengi, an augury is made with an areca blossom, as in menyarung, to determine the suitability of continuing with the cure in a menyarung ceremony. Menyarung may not occur without holding mengadengi first, nor may menyarung proceed directly on the heels of mengadengi.

The cost for holding the ceremony is quite considerable. In one case I studied, requirements were worked out at a meeting held beforehand with the baliens who had been contracted to undertake it. The family was obliged to provide 55 pounds of rice, three small knives (parang or *anak basi*), three chickens, one ceramic jar, three bowls, forty bamboo sticks filled with glutinous rice, and eight eggs, as well as small fish. To raise this capital, the patient's family worked together by tapping 90 pounds of rubber latex.

The Meanings of Objects and Payments

Six categories of objects used in the balien system may be distinguished, based on how they are contributed, used, and disposed of following use in the ceremony.

1. instruments specific to baliens and their ceremonies: stones (batu kait, batu bubut), medicinal oil (polek mo), hook-tipped pole (pangait), and awl (wase).
2. accoutrements specific to the balien: uniform (baju kalawat) and bracelets (tauning).
3. other objects used by the balien but not specific to balien work: cloths, containers (taengen and baranai), bowls, medicinal herbs, and sword.
4. materials obtained and objects prepared specifically for use in the ceremonies: live chicken (to be slaughtered), liquor, rice, bala buloh, leaf offerings, cordyline and other leaves, headdresses, bamboo sticks filled with glutinous rice, eggs, areca blossoms, sweets (sensagun), figurines (sulekale), containers for food offerings, kalangkang and decorations, decorated sun hat, and buluh ayu (decorated bamboo pole). Raw materials are provided by the client, though baliens may contribute labor in preparing them.
5. other objects used but not consumed: ceramic bowls, woven rice container, antique women's clothing on display, percussion instruments, and trays, all provided by the client.
6. payments to the balien (including food displayed in the ceremonies): rice, knives, cloths, bowls, ceramic jars, bamboo sticks filled with glutinous rice, sweets, live chickens, or cash equivalents. In addition, the first time a balien conducts some ceremonies she/he must be presented with a certain specially crafted instrument (e.g., a pangait tip) or an accoutrement (e.g., cloth—kain burih).

Some of these categories overlap. Payments to the balien (category 6) include some materials prepared for use in the ceremonies (category 4) as well as some instruments (category 1) and other objects (category 3). While the buluh ayu is listed in category 4 as an object prepared for the ceremony, it is also an instrument of the balien (category 1), though it is not retained by the balien or used ever again.

Some of the instruments and accoutrements are presented by clients, marking the progress of the balien's career. However, these are payments and not gifts, and they do not signify any special binding relationship between the client and the balien. Other items are prepared by or on behalf of the balien (e.g., by the husband or another family member), such as the wooden pole used for the pangait. The blouse (baju kalawat) is worked on by several baliens who are paid for their work. Other accoutrements are provided by the individual balien without being given by a client.

Very different from all these objects are the balien's stones and oil (polek mo), which are not considered manmade at all; rather, they are believed to have come into being in the course of the ceremony, by virtue of the baliens' abilities to see and catch spirits. These objects are not exchangeable or easily replaceable. In Annette Weiner's terms, they are "symbolically dense—so dense with cultural meaning and value that others have difficulty prying these treasures from their owners" (Weiner 1994: 394). Examples of irreplaceable objects are a monarch's crown (Weiner 1994: 394) or a wedding ring (Baudrillard 1981). Such objects should not be alienated from their owners.

The stones belong definitively to an individual balien; those with individual names have unique significance, and they are never given away or exchanged; but they cannot be equated with Weiner's (1992) "inalienable possessions," not because they cannot be alienated (Weiner's point is that such possessions can be) but because there is no procedure for disposing of or inheriting them. People keep stones left by deceased family members rather than discarding them, but these are scarcely "family jewels" or heirlooms to be handed down in perpetuity. A balien acquires his or her own stones through initiation rather than from a predecessor. Admittedly, a balien's loss of stones—especially the tamang (a balien's tamang is equated with nothing less than that balien's own soul)—would be a traumatic personal loss and would prevent a balien from participating in any of his or her duties. In the event that a balien is alienated from his or her own stones, they may be replaced, but only through reinitiation.

Jean Baudrillard mentions one special sense of the notion of an "object." This is "an object of psychic investment and fascination, of passion and projection—qualified by its exclusive relation with the subject, who then cathects it as if it were his own body" (Baudrillard 1981: 63–34). Among the instruments of the balien, the individually named stones seem to fit this special sense of "object"—but not entirely, for Baudrillard goes on to add that this kind of object is "useless and sublime" (1981: 63–64). It is not instrumental at all; it is purely projective, an object of beauty, for contemplation and perhaps display. The balien's stones, on the contrary, epitomize the balien's instrumentality.

No piece of the balien's equipment is totally inalienable; even a balien's stones could be used by another balien. The pangait may also be used by another balien. Like the stones, it is personal property, though the balien's sentimental attachment to it is undoubtedly weaker. In contrast to these instruments, the balien's accoutrements are not "objects" in Baudrillard's special sense, and they may be replaced without the owner feeling a sense of loss.

Things used in the ceremonies may be displayed, consumed in the course of the ceremony, or given as payment to the balien. Apart from useful consumable goods such as rice, certain durable objects or tokens accrue to the balien as compensation for participating in the rituals. These payments are not commercial transactions but are rather ceremonially prescribed ritual transactions. Thus the tokens are "special purpose monies," in George Dalton's (1967: 254) terms, because they perform certain noncommercial money uses. These tokens may be exchanged or used in payment, but they need not circulate further. Of course such objects have many uses and values apart from the healing situation. But, like objects given in paying brideprice or adat fines, payment for healing is traditionally expressed by the presentation of a few objects customarily associated with the particular domain.[11] Some of the object tokens given to the balien are the same as those used to pay for treatment with antidote oils—cloth, plates, rice, and knives.[12] They seem to go together in a configuration as payments for medicine. The constellation of goods associated with healing suggests a distinctive economic organization specific to the domain of healing. Ideally, payments for treatment are moneyless transactions, but they have been "rationalized" to the extent that money is substituted for objects. (In the case of medicinal oils, owners of medicine may require payment in money in addition to customary objects.)

Important objects used in the menyarung ceremony, such as sarung ase (rice hat), kalangkang (offering tray), and mayang pinang (areca blossom), have no use to the balien following initiation but are kept in perpetuity as mementos and may not be discarded. For a while they are displayed on walls and posts or suspended from rafters and may eventually be stored in lofts. The kalangkang may be lent to neighbors holding the mengadengi ceremony, who keep it until it is demanded by another party.

Prominent among the materials displayed in ceremonies—and later devolving onto the balien—is rice.[13] For subsistence horticulturalists such as the Taman, rice is equated with capital and commercial transaction. Before the use of money in commercial trade, it is probable that rice was used generally as an instrument of transaction. Rice historically has provided the Taman and other shifting cultivators of Borneo with their main source of disposable income (Sather 1994: 128). Prestige goods would be obtained by selling surplus rice. Rice surpluses would also be consumed at feasts (*gawa'*) that increased the prestige and spiritual merit of the sponsors.

The symbolic meaning of rice transcends its economic value, since the Taman subsistence economy is focused on rice cultivation. Spirits, gods, and goddesses (most importantly Grandmother Ambong, the goddess of rice) must be propitiated in rituals to bless rice harvests and ensure success and wealth. Clifford Sather (1994: 130) has described the supreme importance of rice to the Iban, whose worldview is similar to that of the Taman: "Rice represents a transubstantiation of the ancestors, a direct physical embodiment of their continuing presence in the living world." For the Taman as for the Iban, rice has a soul and is the principal symbol of the continuity of life.

The display of large amounts of uncooked rice in ritual is in traditional terms analogous to a ceremonial display of money or gold, that is, a display of capital and wealth, which may have a beneficial and propitiatory effect in attracting spirits and also serve as a status display to the audience. The rice displayed in the balien ceremonies is given in payment to the baliens, as is the other food used in the ceremony. But unlike the other food, the rice is not displayed all at once; it is measured out incrementally over the course of the ceremony, doled out like the cups of liquor given to each balien before dancing. The movement of rice from a basket onto plates and finally into a second basket measures the progress of the ritual and also suggests that fresh rice must be used each time the dance is performed. This aspect of the ritual also suggests that the payment to the balien is calculated as a bowl of rice for each dance performed.

Customary requirements regarding payments to the balien, though rigid in theory, may in practice be negotiable. They may be liberally interpreted or waived, depending on the inclination of the balien. An object used for a ceremony may be returned instead of kept. Substitutions may be made: For example, if a chicken required in compensation of the balien's work is not available (as is commonly the case) Rp 500 may be substituted; Rp 100 may be given instead of a knife; and other exchange values are accepted as the equivalent of bowls or ceramic jars. Furthermore, the balien may not insist that payment for services be settled on the spot by the client; rather, it is understood that the client pledges to pay it. The balien may, however, decline to serve unless payment is made. In these cases the balien can demand immediate payment by saying that it is required because of custom or that spirits insist on it.

Conclusion

The notion that there is a particular technique or state of consciousness unique to shamanism is an overgeneralization. It is necessary to deconstruct and problematize the various somatic states involved in trance as a bodily experience, as Thomas Csordas (1993) has done. Csordas refers to existential psychiatry and phenomenological philosophy in developing an anthropology of experience and embodiment, based on the premise that perception is situated in a culturally constructed world. Csordas criticizes conventional anthropological descriptions of trance and ritual healing for taking the notion of "trance" as a given, without describing in more detail the sensations felt by healers in relation to their patients.

> A conventional anthropology of ritual healing would say simply that the healer goes into trance, assuming trance to be a unitary variable or a kind of black box factored into the ritual equation, and perhaps assuming that somatic manifestations are epiphenomena of trance. The analysis would go no further than informants' reports that these epiphenomena "function" as a confirmation of divine power and healing. (Csordas 1993: 140)

Csordas's analysis of "somatic modes of attention" as "culturally elaborated attention *to* and *with* the body in the immediacy of an intersubjective milieu" (1993: 139) is relevant to the present discussion because the balien uses three different techniques to work with spirits in the ceremonies. These are (1) a clinical technique, in which the balien feels the disease and asks questions of the patient to construct a history. In this phase, the stones are used with herbal medicines; (2) a seance technique, in which the balien sees, hears, and communicates with spirits, employing soul journeying. This technique also enables the balien to see the patient's imperiled soul. Stones are used along with the pangait and medicine (polek mo); and (3) a conjuring technique, in which spirits are invited with offerings. The pangait is used with the stones to convey the balien's voice, but in the menyarung ceremony a decorated bamboo pole (buluh ayu) may be used instead.

There is a clear hierarchy of therapies in Taman balienism; only at the lowest level do subtleties of clinical interpretation come into play. This therapy, the bubut, is the most elementary of balien ceremonies, and may be contrasted with the more advanced seance and stone-catching cures. Bubut therapy frames all balien ceremonies. Clinical interaction, including the clinical-type examination of the patient's body, is confined to this phase of therapy. The signs interpreted in the balien's other ceremonies originate in nonclinical sources: seances, oracles, and auguries.

Whatever is withdrawn from the body is believed to be determined by the spirits rather than by the balien. The point of view underlying balien cures accepts the premise that the objects removed by the balien reflect the nature of the sick person's illness. Because of the balien's relationship with spirits, initiated by the spirit and then altered through menyarung, the balien is able to use stones to feel and remove disease and to interpret illness. By simulating the removal of a certain kind of object from a certain part of the body with a certain stone, the balien is in effect making a specific interpretation of the disease. The stones used to massage the body and the pebbles and splinters that are magically removed constitute a nonverbal medical discourse.

The hierarchical scale of the ceremonies contributes to their "ritual involution," a term coined by Stanley Tambiah (1985: 153). Each successive ceremony incorporates all the previous ones. Each is more complex and takes longer to perform. Each involves more elaborate ceremonialism and material provisioning. Finally, each increasingly advanced ceremony attracts a larger audience. While there may be no witnesses to a bubut, a large cross-section of the village populace may be present for a menyarung.

Bubut is the only ceremony conducted in the balien's residence. In all of the more advanced ceremonies, the balien is brought to the patient's home. A different circumstance prevails in that fewer baliens are qualified and more than one is required. In these cases it is often necessary to recruit at least one balien from outside the village. This increase in the required number of baliens as a function of ritual involution reaches its zenith in the menyarung ceremony, in which up to ten baliens may perform.

Notes

1. The reader may want to compare Harrisson's (1965: 260-264) summary of the balien's ceremonial system, which is quite different from mine. Harrisson did not directly observe any balien ceremonies since he conducted no fieldwork in any Taman villages, but only interviewed three Taman men in the Sarawak Museum. Under the circumstances, and given the intricacy of the balien system, it is not surprising that his account of it is utterly confused.

2. The notion that one reaches the spirit world by means of a ladder is general in shamanism. In the words of Eliade (1964: 487), there are "countless examples of shamanic ascent to the sky by means of a ladder." Besides actual ladders, Eliade cites several analogues: "rainbow, bridge, stairs, vine, cord, 'chain of arrows,' mountain, etc., etc." (1964: 492). Eliade's view that the ladder connects "heaven and earth" does not correctly explain the use of the pangait in the mangait ceremony, since the spirits being contacted in this case are not located on a celestial plane but rather in an unseen dimension of the everyday, terrestrial world.

3. It seems unlikely that the balien keeps together in a single carrying basket (taengen) all the stones (minus the bubut stones) collected on his or her behalf during the menyarung and mengadengi ceremonies. In the menyarung ceremony alone, seven baliens each collecting six stones per day for four days would produce 168 stones. Even if many of these are small, together they would make a very heavy weight to carry around.

4. The names of the patient's older brothers.

5. Goodman (1990) has pointed out that certain postures such as crouching (Goodman calls it the "bear posture") are universal to shamanism and are conducive to trance, as she and "some interested volunteers" (1990:19) found out through experimentation. The posture in which the foot is placed over the sword corresponds to what Goodman calls the "Tennessee diviner" posture.

6. The spirit being addressed by the balien is called Isen, a respectful term

used to address the parents of one's children's spouses. The use of this term signifies that the balien's relationship to the spirit world is one not only of warmth but also of respect. The balien uses this term because she is asking a favor of the spirit: the release of the patient's soul.

7. The balien refers to the patient as grandchild (*anak ampu*) so that the spirit will take pity on him or her.

8. Later that night another balien agreed with me that it made no sense for the child to be treated by a balien. It seems that this was a final, desperate attempt to cure the boy and that the balien ceremony was inappropriate as treatment for the illness. The boy died three days later, having been taken to his parents' village upstream the night after the mangait service.

9. Harrisson (1965: 260–261) mentions this term and provides an account of the ceremony. *Maniang* is a general term for the balien's healing seances, and *aso* refers to the daytime.

10. King (1985: 231) translates *wase* as "adze," as does Diposiswoyo (1985: 317). Judging from Diposiswoyo's illustration of this implement (1985: 285), however, the instrument used by the balien in the malai ceremony is an adze head (*mata uase*), though it is too small to be fitted to a handle and function as an agricultural tool. It is specially forged for the balien, who refers to it as *kangkuang basi* (iron drum), for use in the ceremony. The Taman also call it *penyalak*. Harrisson (1965: 260) translates wase (*wasay*) as "hatchet."

11. A good example is the required payment to the balien of a bowl for having her stones carried across the river. Such a payment is not justified in terms of the balien's work. Rather, it is dictated by custom.

12. Payments for treatment with oils, however, also include other objects not associated with balienism: sewing needles and thread. Clearly, these objects go together, but the reason they are selected as tokens of payment is not clear to me, other than the fact that needles are "fed" to oils to sustain them. For a discussion of the payments and of the commodity status of poisons and antidotes see Bernstein 1993b: 17–19.

13. Gifts of rice are also sometimes presented by extended kin to help the patient's household bear the cost of more elaborate ceremonies such as malai.

7

Balienism in Society

This chapter considers the balien's profession in the context of social and psychological integration. While the primary focus is the institutionalization of knowledge and its social ramifications, these issues are ultimately inseparable from issues of the "internalization" of the profession as an expression of the self (De Vos 1990). In this chapter I focus on aspects of the self and identity, such as gender, chronic illness, and social adjustment, in relationship to being a balien. I also address the question of the mental normality of the balien. First, it is important to determine the place of the baliens and their ceremonies in Taman society.

The Balien's Profession as
Organized Activity and Social Collectivity

The balien's task of curing people shares certain characteristics of professional occupations, and it can be likened to one. One way in which balienism is institutionalized as a profession is that it is treated as a kind of work that must be compensated in esteem of the service rendered. Thus, it differs from both Sakalava spirit-mediumship in Madagascar (Sharp 1990) and Wana shamanism in Sulawesi (Atkinson 1989: 273), in which payments are intended to benefit the spirit-familiars rather than the practitioners.

The work of the balien can also be contrasted with other Taman ceremonies for which the performer is not paid, such as offerings (*tentalayong*). In traditional legal cases, too, the person adjudicating the case (normally the headman) is not customarily paid, although he may require a volume of liquor from the disputants, as well as food, coffee, and other provisions to be consumed during the session.

Another way in which balienism resembles a profession is that baliens are characterized by a monopoly on special knowledge and practices. Their domain of knowledge is not common to other members of society, and no one other than a balien is legitimately able to conduct any of its practices. Baliens also control the entry of new members into their group.

Finally, baliens serve a distinctive need in Taman society: Their role is certainly a "service-oriented" and "consultative" one, to borrow the terms Eliot Freidson (1970) used in describing medicine as a profession. By performing their ceremonies, baliens affect the social order in a way functionally similar to that of medical personnel: by interpreting and treating illness.

However, there are limits to the validity of any comparison between balienism and "professions," as the term is applied in modern postindustrial society. The balien's work is not a full-time occupation, and its rewards do not enable anyone to make a living. Perhaps more important, the balien does not have a distinct relationship to social and economic power, and the balien group does not mobilize its activities to function as a base of power for its members.

While the comparison between the balien's profession and that of trained medical practitioners—especially doctors—may be intriguing, it is not altogether apt. Like doctors, baliens possess special knowledge, but it is not of a biomedical order. To understand the nature of the balien's profession, it is more illuminating to situate it in the context of the healing practices of ritual, magical, and religious specialists, particularly those who, like the balien, may be called shamans.

Balienism as Magic and Thaumaturgy

In contrasting magic and religion, William Goode (1951) says that magic is characterized by a concrete specificity of goals, and that the client approaches the professional as a private individual rather than as a representative of some group. While most balien ceremonies have fairly specific goals, the purpose of the menyarung ceremony, as well as the illness and other problems leading up to it, seems vaguer, and more global. Becoming a balien seems to entail the recognition of a change in one's whole way of being. Also, while it is true that balien ceremonies do not treat the society as a whole, they do cure whole families as a single unit.

Emile Durkheim (1976: 44–45) makes some valid points about the sociological difference between religion and magic.

> The magician has a clientele and not a Church, and it is very possible that his clients have no other relations between each other or even do not know each other; even the relations which they have with him are generally accidental and terminal; they are just like those of a sick man with his physician. The official and public character with which he is sometimes invested changes nothing in this situation; the fact that he works openly does not unite him more regularly or more durably to those who have recourse to his services. It is true that in certain cases magicians form societies among themselves. . . . But . . . these associations are in no way indispensable to

the workings of the magic. The magician has no need of uniting himself to his fellows to practice his art.

In Durkheim's view, "religion is inseparable from the idea of a Church," by which he means "a moral community formed by all the believers in a single faith, laymen as well as priests. But magic lacks any such community." *"There is no Church of magic."* In other words, religion is socially organized. What about magic? Durkheim seems to deny that it is socially organized, though he does consider the notion of a "society of magic":

> When these societies of magic are formed, they do not include all the adherents to magic, but only magicians; the laymen . . . for whose profit the rites are celebrated, in fine, those who represent the worshipers in regular cults, are excluded. Now the magician is for magic what the priest is for religion, but a college of priests is not a church, any more than a religious congregation which should devote itself to some particular saint in the shadow of a cloister would be a particular cult. (Durkheim 1976: 44–45)

Balienism is more than a number of operators administering their cures individually. The "society of magic," to use Durkheim's phrase, is organized in a consequential way among the Taman. In Max Weber's (1964: 324ff.) terms, balienism is grounded in legitimacy. The Malay dukun may well correspond to Durkheim's stereotype of the magician as a "recluse from society," but not the balien.

Balienism is first of all a set of organized and purposeful activities, complex procedures governed by rules. But it is more, because the only people who can carry them out are those who have been ritually inducted into the group of personnel. There is a hierarchy not only to activities but to personnel. Personnel are set apart by their distinctive uniforms and instruments. Perhaps most important, they are thought to be united in having suffered afflictions from spirits, and their lives are considered to be different from those of other people in that they are able not only to perceive spirits but initiate contact with them. They are linked together in an association that includes spirits of deceased practitioners of their work.

Unfortunately, there exists no well-defined vocabulary to characterize the organization of personnel in the balien system. At first I considered proposing that they constitute a "healing cult," but while the term "cult" in some ways suggests the phenomenon I am talking about, it also implies worship and devotion, as well as deviation from the prevailing belief system. I. M. Lewis (1971: 88–89), for example, writes that women's healing cults are ostensibly therapeutic but that "reports of the elaborate, if furtive, rituals involved" indicate that their underlying significance is as "clandestine religion" promulgating a subversive "feminist sub-culture." The balien system is deeply grounded in Taman society's traditional cultural belief system, and should not be confused with any of the affliction cults enumerated by Lewis.

Also, the term "magic" is too broad to provide much insight into either the practice or social organization of balienism. Allan Young (1975) writes of magic as a "quasi-profession," but this, too, is not very specific. Instead, I use the term "thaumaturgy," a word found in Bryan Wilson's *Magic and the Millennium* (1973), meaning "wonder-working, conjuring, working miracles or wonders." Balienism is, then, a thaumaturgical association. In the context of Wilson's study, it should be pointed out that balienism is nonprophetic, nonmillennial, nonmessianic, and nondenominational; it is not even a "movement."

Shamans and Shaman/Healers

Michael Winkelman's (1992) useful distinction between shamans and shaman/healers points to evidence that thaumaturgical associations such as that of the balien are socially organized. The classic or primal shaman is Siberian, Central Asian, or Eskimo (e.g., the Tungus *saman,* the Chukchee *ene nilit,* and the Eskimo *angakoq*), but others, such as the Paiute *puha* or *puhaba,* would also be considered true shamans. The shaman is a charismatic leader and has high social status, though he or she lacks high economic status. Shamans and shaman/healers differ mainly in their social organization. Shamans generally carry out professional duties without assistance from other shamans, and are generally trained by another shaman acting alone. Although shamans do not have professional groups, they may engage in contests or other forms of competition. Shamans have individual teachers, learn incidentally from observation, or are taught directly by the spirits (Winkelman 1992: 50). Unlike the shaman/healer, who acts only at a client's request, and within that client's group, the shaman can also work for his or her own entire local community and can use both malevolent and beneficent magic. The social position of the shaman appears to be determined by the fact that the shaman complex is associated with nomadism and hunter-gatherer subsistence; in fact, the shaman is the only kind of magicoreligious practitioner found in such societies, according to Winkelman. However, the shaman complex is not completely correlated with low sociopolitical integration or minimal fixity of residence (Winkelman 1992: 49).

Staying with Winkelman's typology, the shaman/healer, of which type the balien is representative, is generally found in societies that have more than one kind of magicoreligious practitioner; however, Winkelman points out that the shaman/healer is found at all levels of social and political integration. Shaman/healers have a higher degree of professional social organization and more intensive involvement in group activities than do shamans; these include collective ceremonies and training by groups rather than by individuals. Shaman/healers may have joint ceremonies, formal group activities, and may formally acquire status through ceremonial initiation. Shaman/healers are predominantly male, though females are allowed to occupy the status. Shaman/healers do not have high status socially or economically, in part because of the dominance of priests. They are part-time specialists, supporting themselves through subsistence or other remunerative work. They lack high sociopolitical power, though they may act as diviners and can exercise charismatic power if there is no priest in the society. Their moral status is considered predominantly benevolent, but it is recognized that they can use their powers to cause harm. Shaman/healers are taught by a practitioner group. Generally they enter the role voluntarily, though illness or involuntary visions can also be the basis of selection. Relations with spirits, mainly animal spirits and other minor spirits, are the main sources of their power. Shaman/healers generally command spirits and do not use propitiation. They are thought to be able to transform themselves into animals. Besides their relationships with spirits, the shaman/healer's techniques include rubbing; massaging; cleansing of wounds; application of herbal medicine; object extraction (sleight of hand); spells and charms; exuvial, imitative, and manipulative techniques; and exorcism and other spirit control (Winkelman 1992: 56).

The Social Organization of the Balien Association

The personnel and doctrines of the thaumaturgical association come to the fore in the menyarung ceremony. Initiation is carried out by a quorum including many proven baliens from within the local community (and usually some from outside the community as well), but the approval of the souls of revered dead baliens (*balien tutun*), indicated through the areca blossom augury, is needed to fully confirm induction. Apart from this ceremony, however, balienism is weakly institutionalized. Leadership by senior baliens who are well versed in chants is tacit. The great majority of members are women with little if any potential for (or apparent interest in) wielding political or economic power. The rare male baliens are withdrawn people.

There is a great difference between baliens and other curers in the village. Certain people in the village have an abiding interest in collecting medicines either to protect and/or medicate their own family or to use them for profit. There is virtually no interest in using the medicines altruistically. If a medicine is used to cure people, the payment is said to be determined by the medicine and not by the owner's pecuniary interests. However, there is no imperative to cure because there is no need to publicize one's possession of a medicine. For the balien, there is this imperative.

The technical medical knowledge of the balien, embedded in a discourse of stones, in part consists of the technique of palpating the patient's body. The stones used to remove disease and the objects removed specify the nature of the disease both concretely and verbally, as described above. The baliens who work together in an initiation ceremony collect that novice's stones, and baliens who cooperatively cure a patient know the names of each other's stones. For example, a balien leading a chant will name the tamang (stone double) of her partner, saying that that stone longs for a spirit.

To what extent does the thaumaturgical association of baliens function as a corporation or organization? Weber (1964:145–152) has maintained that the essential characteristic of any corporate group or organization is that at least one person exercises authority and provides leadership. According to Weber, a corporate group is governed by some system of order, and provision must be made for the enforcement of rules. By this definition the balien association is not an organization, since political and administrative power is not organized among its members. There is no living leader of the baliens, and rules are not administered within the group; order is maintained through other means. The association is held together by customary practices and equipment, mystified occult knowledge, experiences of involuntary and unwelcome contact with spirits, a common sense of affliction, and techniques for perceiving, contacting, and manipulating spirits within altered states of consciousness. Thus, the balien association does not fit into any of Lewis's (1971) categories that would explain socially organized ecstasy, since it is not concerned with issues of morality, leadership, power, or social position, either in the content of its ceremonies or in the consequences for its members.

Let us consider the social organization of balienism: their groupings, forms of association and interaction, and common activities. My study of several Taman villages suggests that baliens do not closely associate with one another informally. People associate mainly with other people in their family and longhouse or other local group. Baliens maintain the same group of intimates—the kindred—after their initiation as they did before. Even when visiting other villages or more distant places, it is invariably someone from within the kindred who is called upon for hospitality. Baliens do not have any regularly scheduled meetings. Their sole purpose in coming together is to professionally execute a task, namely, the cure of a sickness. The matter of scheduling is the responsibility of the client (meaning the patient and his or her family members who contract and pay for the service) and not the baliens.

The balien's legitimacy—his or her socially recognized ability to cure—is based solely on an ability to see and feel spirits. Baliens may be contrasted with healers in those societies, like the Bagobo (Payne 1985), who enter healing work because of a sense of vocation. Unlike Bagobo healers, who are expected to have pure motives and to have internalized a sense of pity, baliens are not required to present themselves as selflessly devoted to the care of their patients. Furthermore, it is not the place of the baliens to provide commentary but only to execute the ceremony according to the dictates of tradition. It is the spirits, especially the spirits of the deceased baliens, who judge the success of the ceremony, and the baliens who interpret their messages, tending to view the ceremonies as successful. No inductee ever fails to be initiated.

A balien treating a patient would not say that the person cannot be cured, nor would a balien cancel a healing ceremony that had begun after receiving signs from the spirits to that effect. Instead, the balien would complete the ceremony and advise the patient to visit a doctor and get an injection. On one point balien ideology is clear: Baliens themselves accept no responsibility for failures. Curing is viewed as the beneficence of God or the spirit, and the balien, like any other healer, is merely a helper.

Informants said that novices worked under the supervision of senior ranking baliens. Less experienced baliens are in fact deputized in assignments, but there is no critical assessment of the balien's work. Baliens work cooperatively in several therapies, dividing tasks as appropriate and discussing the meanings of oracles to arrive at a consensus. There are no subspecialties of balienism. What may appear to be specialization is a result of the fact that many baliens are limited to performing only the simpler ceremonies.[1]

Furthermore, there is no external control on the balien's progress. Although there are many baliens, there is often a pressing need for any available balien because villagers are dispersed in their cultivated fields. Because there is a considerable demand for the balien's services, it is not possible for a balien to thwart another's professional advancement. Since a client may choose any capable and available balien he or she wants, it is not possible for a single balien, or baliens from one segment of society, to become disproportionately powerful. The leading baliens in the society (*balien sarin*) are far more interested in their families and private lives than in doctrine or control. There is no evidence of any but the most casual patronage of baliens.

The Status of the Balien

Baliens do not have higher status than ordinary people, but they do have a special role.[2] Among nonindustrialized peoples such as the Taman there exist few specialized roles other than political functionaries (chieftain, complex head, headman, and deputy headman). Most ceremonial work can be and is performed by nonspecialist functionaries. Each village has teachers, but these are often outsiders (see Bernstein 1990), as are the two medical aides stationed in Taman villages. Shopkeepers also have a significant role. Although several villages have churches, and a few Taman people are able to lead religious services, professional religious personnel are all outsiders. The role of the balien, in effect, is one of the few truly specialized positions within Taman society, along with the headman and elders capable of functioning as councillors. But being a balien does not affect one's social status in a general sense, unlike possessing a school diploma, holding some official position, or owning a shop. Little if any social power resides in the balien thaumaturgical association. More than advancing one's position of status, being a balien can benefit persons who have difficulties in social or psychological adjustment by providing them a new sense of belonging. It must be remembered that the functioning balien is an individual cured of a malfunction that has been labeled an illness. This recovered sense of belonging is essential to the healing process, as George De Vos (1980: 215) has pointed out: "The healer is at best able to remove the causes of deviancies so that the individual can become part of the society. Healing behavior can be seen, therefore, as a ritual of incorporation or restitution by which the malfunctioning is cured; the handicap is overcome so that the individual can assume an appropriate role in the society."

Since most people do not occupy other specialized roles that could conflict with the role of the balien, I should mention the case of a certain headman about whom a rumor spread that he was planning to be initiated as a balien. The man staunchly denied this to me, saying that the balien's role was incompatible with his role as headman. How, he asked, could he preside authoritatively over disputes if he had to heal (bubut) all the people coming to his door? He was describing the balien's work as a career, a full-time role and responsibility, not as a treatment for persistent illness.

Baliens are not degraded or despised; unlike participants in cults and spirit possession and mediumship elsewhere in the world (see Lewis 1971), they are not considered to be beyond the pale of normal society. Despite their intimacy with the supernatural, baliens are not feared by laymen, nor are they considered in any way to be weird or dangerous. Far from being considered deviant, they are thought to have overcome their troubles in culturally appropriate ways and can cure people because of their special status.

Ranking

Baliens may be ranked according to their ability to serve in and lead healing ceremonies, the virtuosity of their chanting, and their ability to perform wondrous feats in healing ceremonies. The actual ranking of baliens is not absolute or unanimously agreed upon but is personal and possibly idiosyncratic. Moreover, it is considered slightly unseemly to compare baliens. Nevertheless, there are definite classes of baliens.

The Taman distinguish between more and less accomplished baliens. There is a clear gradation of the ceremonies, and the ability of a particular balien to perform (and especially lead) them determines her or his level of accomplishment. The honorific title for the most prominent baliens is balien sarin. The term "balien tutun" is also heard, mainly in the chants, in which the most revered and skilled of the dead baliens are commemorated: Their names are recited as they are invited to participate and help deliberate in determining the origin and required cure of a disease. *Tutun,* from *tutu,* meaning "highest or topmost" (King 1985: 231), describes a balien whose diagnoses and procedures are always correct. The calling of the dead baliens suggests a continuum of "terrestrial" and "celestial" baliens, to use the terms of Penelope Graham (1987) in her study of Iban shamanism. By calling the celestial baliens by name, the terrestrial baliens show deference while indicating that they work together. The celestial baliens, especially Grandmother Siunsun Amas, the patron spirit or ancestress of the baliens, establish the procedures. They give order and structure to the profession of the balien by judging the balien's work and by giving or withholding blessings for success. In each of the balien's treatments, an offering is made to the celestial baliens so that they will participate in curing the patient.

"Balien sarin" is the honorific term used for great baliens, baliens of high rank who are knowledgeable about all aspects of the balien's craft and are capable of leading complex ceremonies such as menindoani and menyarung. It refers to those who lead the menyarung and hence are considered teachers as well as to baliens who are always called upon to participate in the menyarung ceremony and who, in the words of informants, may not be left behind. The term "sarin" appears to refer not to a distinct group of baliens but rather to the most senior relatively. The use of this sobriquet seems to be a judgment of quality. One balien said by all to be sarin was unable to lead chants. Because chanting is the major work not only in menyarung and mengadengi but in lesser ceremonies as well, she has a deputizing role whenever she works in concert with other baliens. But because of her experience, seniority, and popularity, she is indisputably sarin.

There is a lore about the great baliens of former times having performed miraculous cures, such as healing a person whose body had been severed in two. This lore is indicative of the balien's mystique of esotericism.

Esotericism

Esotericism is unquestionably a part of what separates the balien from the nonbalien. The balien's specialized domain is rarefied. Furthermore, there is deliberate mystification in the use of sleight of hand to catch stones and remove objects with stones. These stones are mystified by the baliens and used as magical objects. If the stones are used by nonbaliens, their magical properties cannot be realized.

An enlightened balien can supposedly see into the future, although not necessarily with clarity. Once a balien examining the areca blossom cracked open at the conclusion of a menyarung ceremony said, "Perhaps someone among us will depart soon." The balien did not announce this, and most people in attendance could not hear her words, but less than a year later one of the baliens who participated in the ceremony died.

I sometimes heard incredible stories about the powers of the baliens. For example, I was told that if a balien dives into water to retrieve the soul of a person, he or she comes out of the water dry. The following is another example of the balien's mystery. In the words of a Taman man:

> When the balien dances with the bowl on her head, it never falls off, no matter how much she moves. But if a balien can't be cured and [is destined to] die, the plate will fall off. This happened to Payung when she performed at someone's place. The plate fell off her head and broke during the ceremony, and she died about a year later.

Who Becomes a Balien?

In principle, any person could be afflicted by dawawa jalu or pais layu-layu and be forced to become a balien. Yet certain conditions seem to predispose a person to enter this occupation. The factors to be considered are chronic illness, gender, psychological health and normality, and moral and economic support from one's kin group. Except for the last of these, all could be seen to be mainly internal issues of identity and adjustment. However, all have a social component.

Chronic Illness

Chronic illness is the most commonly named factor predisposing a person to become a balien. While the syndromes suffered by the balien candidate should be regarded as hysterical (see Chapter 5), these syndromes frequently include nonpsychogenic disorders that may precede the other abnormalities. Yet serious chronic illness seems to be neither a sufficient nor necessary predicate of the balien's vocation. Certain baliens were only mildly ill prior to initiation, while other chronically ill people do not consider it a possibility that they will ever become baliens. Nevertheless, a chronically ill person may after some years reach a point at which it becomes necessary to follow the course to initiation. The process, which takes several years, may be seen as a stage of life, and it needs to be examined in a life-course perspective such as that used by the psychologist Daniel Levinson (1978).

Rather than pure chronicity of illness, the determining factor seems to be how the illness responds to efforts by baliens to treat it. Analytically, sickness rather than illness brings people to be treated by baliens into a process that may lead eventually to their being initiated. Sickness is the social enactment of illness through self-presentation in relation to family members, healers, and others. If a person has been successfully cured of all symptoms, there is no motivation for continuing the process toward initiation.

The balien's illnesses, like any illnesses, are socially expressed in sickness, and this suggests a certain incapacity to function properly. But in becoming a balien, a person is never merely the passive subject of the decisions and actions of others. While others may influence the decision to become a balien, the choice is finally up to the individual person.

Gender

The great majority of Taman baliens are women. The Sibau branch of the Taman, including the villages at Sibau Hilir, Sibau Hulu, and Tanjung Lasa, had a population of 2,065 in 1986, including over three hundred non-Taman residents. During the time of my research, there were over twenty baliens (the exact number varied as some baliens died and new ones were initiated). Three of these were men, and of those, only one was a practitioner. The second male balien, whom I never met, was too old to practice, and the third had discontinued his practice, saying that since another man had been initiated he felt there was no need for him to continue as a male balien. In Semangkok on the Mendalam River, of a population of 380 there were eight initiated baliens, of whom one was a man. Among the Kapuas Taman, too, there were far more female than male baliens. Considering that it is not the entire population that is prone to becoming a balien but only mature adults, it can be estimated that odds of a woman becoming a balien sometime in her life are at least one in twenty. Women are about seven times more likely than men to become baliens; subsequent to initiation, they are significantly more likely to continue to practice and excel at balienism than their male counterparts.

Furthermore, as baliens idealize the legendary ancestress Grandmother Siunsun Amas, it is justifiable to say that the balien is prototypically a woman.[3] Although the thaumaturgical association of baliens is not in absolute terms a "women's cult," since it does not exclude men, it is dominated by women. Women not only lead the services but perform most of the other chores in balien ceremonies, such as filling rice bowls and playing music. However, men tend to lead the convoys escorting the baliens to the site where the patient's soul is caught, put oil on the stones as they are caught, and assist by serving refreshments; men are no less represented in the audiences of balien ceremonies than are women, and—menyarung aside—men seem to be the patients of baliens as often as women.

Winkelman (1992: 45) has provided a correlation of traits associated with magicoreligious occupations that are dominated by men and by women. Winkelman finds those roles occupied exclusively by men to be characterized by extensive sociopolitical power and high socioeconomic status. The practitioner group is hierarchical, with members selected through inheritance, succession, or political action. Power derives from superior gods, and altered states of consciousness are not used. Those roles that are predominantly but not exclusively held by men are very different, though they, too, are characterized by judiciary powers and high socioeconomic status. Those that are predominantly female are characterized by no political power, low socioeconomic status, and little or no control over one's magical power. (Winkelman provides no examples of exclusively female magico-religious occupations.)

Such a pattern supports Robert Winzeler's (1993: xxviii) explanation for the preponderance of female shamans among the Taman: While the role of women as ritual specialists is diminished in Christianity (and also, for that matter, in Judaism and Islam), it remains high in shamanism. Therefore, while men will have other ways to serve as ritual functionaries in introduced religions, "women will turn to the more durable traditions of shamanism," leading to female domination.

Taman people's own explanation for the preponderance of women among baliens is that women's sickness is more often treatable by or fit for balien treatment than is men's. Women's chronic illnesses, therefore, are more prone to be cast as pais layu-layu than are men's. Men's illnesses, even when treated as a spirit affliction, are usually either resolved at that stage (in the mengadengi ceremony) or cured by another mode of treatment before reaching the stage of initiation.

Why is balienism primarily a female phenomenon? It is possible, following the proposals of certain feminist social scientists (e.g., Epstein 1970), to look at differences in the life experiences of men and women to account for the difference in likelihood. Men in Borneo generally have the opportunity to travel to other parts of Borneo, where they are introduced to a variety of work experiences and cultural possibilities that are alternatives to the ones with which they grew up. Starting in their youth, males have the opportunity to go to Sarawak, where they can escape the confines of village life. (These trips are idealized by Taman youths.) Adult men also occasionally go there to work, invariably leaving their wives and children behind, and sometimes returning years later with new wives. Women, however, are rarely able to travel long distances and may be subject to different temptations than men. Staying behind in the village, it is possible for them to get involved in extramarital affairs despite the highly punitive disincentives of customary law.

But differences in life experiences between males and females are not sufficient to explain differences between them in patterns of spirit disturbance, reinterpretation of illness, and balien initiation. Instead, we must consider the power asymmetry between the sexes (Rancour-Laferriere 1985: 275–286), specifically the universal associations in sexuality whereby "male" is equated with "dominance" and "female" with "subordination."[4] Daniel Rancour-Laferriere cites Helene Deutsch's (Deutsch 1944, I: 280) statement that "activity is the share of a man, passivity that of a woman," but he goes on to mention her important caveat: "Passivity does not mean apathy or lack of sexual energy." "Female sexual energy may in fact be very high in Deutsch's scheme" (Rancour-Laferriere 1985: 277). A woman may have high sexual interest and energy yet be very passive sexually. The contradictions between these qualities could lead to conflict, expressed in somatization, fantasy, and the appearance of visions, all of which are interpreted as symptoms of the balien's predisposing illness. Within Taman society, the thaumaturgical association of baliens provides a socially acceptable and culturally meaningful way for women to resolve this conflict between sexual energy and passivity. Since it provides a new role, membership and participation in the association constitute a form of role resolution of psychological conflict, which, in the words of Gananath Obeyesekere (1981: 161), "is one of the most powerful integrative mechanisms in human societies."

The balien's illness as spirit disturbance is explicitly sexualized. Unseen spirits are considered to be part of the real world, and their actuality is taken for granted by most Taman. This is not simply a question of superstition or hallucination. Men believe in their existence at least as much as do women, and both men and women report having personally encountered spirits. But it is mainly women who report being victimized by spirits through seduction. The culturally accepted view of a person's condition before becoming a balien—the view held by the candidate—can be likened to one of femininity: A person is passive, and something happens to her or him. Before becoming a candidate, the person is treated as a medical patient. (The association of initiation with piercing is noteworthy because piercing with hooks similarly puts the person in a passive, or feminine, position.) By becoming a balien she (or he) asserts control over the externalized forces behind apparitions and symptoms. Through initiation, successful baliens achieve mastery: The symptoms of spirit disturbance cease, and spirits that previously caused torment are now put at the balien's disposal.

The balien's destiny is often diagnosed on the basis of a fantasy of being forced to submit sexually. There is substantial psychological evidence that these fantasies are much more common in women than in men. According to Leitenberg and Henning (1995: 482), "The typical female erotic rape fantasy involves imagining a sexually attractive man whose sexual passion is irresistibly stimulated by the woman's sexual attractiveness. In the fantasy, the man uses just enough force to overcome her token resistance and to arouse her sexually." This description corresponds to reports of spirit disturbance among the Taman resulting in both treatment by stone capture (in the mengadengi ceremony) and initiation into the balien group. A possible explanation for the relative preponderance of such fantasies in women is that "a woman raised in an environment with sexual prohibitions can feel blameless if the sexual behavior and stimulation she imagines are not her doing" (Leitenberg and Henning 1995: 483).

There is also cross-cultural and historical evidence that men and women have different somatic styles and that women are relatively more prone than men to express strong emotions through suffering and physical symptoms. As Edward Shorter (1994: 56) has written, "It is likely that both in the past and today women have employed the language of organicity more often than men to cope with unhappiness." Shorter has shown that among both wealthy classes and rural poor, women outnumber men in chronic suffering associated with what modern medicine would label "psychosomatic illness" and "hysteria." In both cases, illness is often a response to "domestic sorrows" and a sense of powerlessness.

Males and females appear to have the same motivations in becoming baliens, although the social forces that bear on the decision tend to have the effect of propelling a woman into balien candidacy and deflecting men from it. The balien, whether male or female, is above all a person who has been cured by coming to terms with the repressed unconscious by projecting threatening thoughts onto external agents who can be related to as friends on an esoteric plane of reality.

Psychological Health and Normalcy

During the performance of the initiation and other spirit-catching ceremonies, baliens sometimes exhibit exaggerated or unusual behavior. They seem to be attuned more to the reality of the ceremony and the spirit world than to the mundane human world. A minority of the baliens are particularly apt to adopt behavior that is humorous to the audience within the ceremony and would be totally inappropriate or even bizarre in other circumstances. The behavior associated with this role allows an individual to express tendencies that cannot otherwise be expressed within this society but that may be widespread in the Taman population.

In Taman ideology, baliens are not inherently different from normal humans, but because of their illness, they are forced to become shamans through an initiation ceremony that transforms them into a special kind of person. Against this, the psychoanalytic anthropologist George Devereux (1980) would argue that baliens, like all shamans, must be psychotic, despite all ideology to the contrary. Devereux's view of shamanism is negative and extreme. He claims that the shaman's initiation does not cure any basic illness but only erects new defenses that eventually become stale. He views the shaman's ability to "feel" disease inside the body as hallucinatory, and consonant with the psychoanalytic definition of psychosis.

Devereux (1980: 4–5) differentiates between external and internal adjustment, making the point that a person may be externally adjusted to his or her society without introjecting its norms. This suggests that conclusions about the normalcy of a person's inner mental functioning cannot be drawn from behavior suggesting social adaptation or maladaptation. Devereux's point that the shaman may be psychopathological despite the appearance of normality and integration in the society is well taken. (Devereux criticizes anthropologists for making clinical types of statements about their informants' personalities without undertaking clinical investigations or having themselves undergone clinical training.) But his argument about the mental abnormality of all shamans is unproved (Kennedy 1973: 1150), and it cannot be concluded from the Taman data that these shamans are necessarily maladjusted. The illnesses of candidate baliens may be pathomimetic adaptations to sexual fantasies. De Vos (1974), contrary to Devereux, is of the opinion that the shaman's predisposing syndrome may be indicative primarily of pathomimesis rather than mental disorder:

> In the shaman, whatever his state of consciousness or self-hypnosis, the behavior becomes socially adaptive as symbolic of religious ecstasy. In pathomimetic phenomena, the possessed individual has somehow learned to manifest convulsions [for example] as a sign that a spirit has entered his body so that communication becomes possible with the supernatural. His manifest behavior may therefore simply be adaptive rather than maladjustive either in structure or function. (De Vos 1974: 563)

Because of the possibility that trances and other shamanistic phenomena mimic mental disorder, more in-depth psychological techniques are necessary to determine whether there is any true psychological pathology in shamanism. A definitive conclusion about the baliens' internal mental adjustment requires clinical studies. The important point here is that baliens have been transformed through initiation precisely to avoid madness (if not other illness or death). Thus, the baliens whose earlier delusions (uncontrolled visions) cease and who are able to harness their imaginative powers in curing ceremonies are well adapted in Taman society as a result of the specialized role available to them.

Moral and Economic Support by Kin Group

Without the resources necessary to hold a menyarung ceremony, the quest to become a balien can be delayed indefinitely. In a previously mentioned case, a woman who had been treated in a night-long stone-catching ceremony was actually willing to continue the course to initiation, but could not do so due to lack of money. As her husband wittily put it, in a clear analogy between the balien's training and formal medical education, she could no more practice balien therapies than a person who had finished one year of lower secondary school (SMP) could work as a doctor. Economic support involving the consolidation or liquidation of resources comes from the patient's family, except in the infrequent case that the patient is a household head. Once definite plans have been made, the larger kindred is approached for aid in holding the ceremony, but the basic provision of rice must be accumulated first by the immediate family. Besides economic support, moral support within the family propels a patient's candidacy. Consensus within the family is sought before a plan is made to continue; in these discussions young people ordinarily defer to elders. In one interesting case, a balien had been widowed for five years at the time of her original illness. Two older men and one older woman in her family suggested that she be initiated. Her children agreed, and three of her cousins raised the capital.

The disturbances leading to balien treatment and ultimately initiation are intricately related to interpersonal problems that occur and are identified within the domestic situation. Therefore, it is unlikely that a person would ever be considered for balien candidacy without the input of his or her domestic family.

Considering the support given by the family, one might ask whether any advantages can accrue to the family of a balien. As we have seen, clients prefer baliens from their own kin group over others. While the family members of a balien are not exempted from a requirement to make customary payments, any fees paid obviously remain within the family. A balien will probably do his or her utmost to cure a family member, but the cure may still not work, and it may be deduced in such cases that the very closeness of the balien's spirit helpers impedes a successful cure. Moreover, advanced cures generally require the work of two baliens. It may be concluded that there are no advantages per se to having a balien in the family.

Balienism as a Career

A number of baliens neither practice curing nor attend ceremonies. Others do not practice because of illness. (Interestingly, a balien's claim of illness is one of the few accepted excuses for not working.) There are those who would say that these baliens are continually sick precisely because they have not accepted the balien's mandate to heal. However, it is noteworthy that most baliens are active, considering that they do not deliberately set about to become baliens. This suggests that there is some correlation between the balien's personality type and the social process whereby illness is reinterpreted as a shamanic destiny.

A balien who is well and does not have another obligation may not decline the invitation to heal unless there is a prohibition by custom. For example, in the case of a recent death a balien will refuse to perform any cures because of danger from spirits of the dead. There seems to be little reluctance to employ untried baliens, but those who are known not to have a penchant for healing cease to be called.

For baliens who are willing to work there is a steady, continual request for cures, and curing becomes a career. Eventually some baliens become known far beyond their own village. A leading balien in Sibau Hilir has been called to cure people in Putussibau, and a young balien has been brought in from Tanjung Lasa to perform her cure in Sibau Hulu, a village in which several baliens are resident. More striking, a certain Embaloh male balien is known to the Sibau Taman, even though his village is at least one day's journey away. But it would be a mistake to think that Taman may be influenced to become baliens by seeing the social recognition achieved by a few baliens or by the relatively small tokens of payment received by baliens.

Even elderly and sickly baliens do some healing. One of the most widely called-upon baliens was a woman in her seventies. Another very decrepit balien did little healing because she was sick most of the time. A distinguished chanter, she was weak and asthmatic, and lacked the energy to do much healing. Within her own longhouse, however, she was frequently pressed into service, curing people using the bubut technique and performing more advanced services when other baliens were not available. She also filled in for baliens who had to cancel their sessions.

Baliens may not work in competition with one another; for example, they may not undercut another's fee or demand a higher fee by claiming to be a superior balien. This is not to deny that there is a potential for individual maneuvering. A balien may say that a more advanced treatment is needed, or may offer to cure the patient with an antidote oil for an additional fee. But those whose interest in medicine is commercial can find profit without becoming baliens, and the path to becoming a balien has no relation to a professional interest in medicine.

By performing and participating in healing ceremonies, an active balien may recoup the initial investment made by the family in the menyarung. Husbands of two female baliens told me that the incomes from their wives' labors had repaid the cost of holding the ceremony and possibly made an income on top of that. Having put large amounts of capital (by local standards) into this ceremony, it is understandable that they were mindful of any return on their investment. But the primary concern of those contributing to the menyarung ceremony, like that of the balien, is the resolution of an intractable illness. Rather than actively contemplating potential earnings, the spouse and other family members of the novice balien hope for a recovery following initiation.

Advancement

Advancement within a profession such as balienism requires a willingness on the part of the practitioner to administer more complex cures and the willingness of a client to commission an inexperienced person. As we have seen, the balien performs ceremonies that she or he is not competent to lead by serving as a deputy. The main factor determining the balien's ability to move to a higher level of achievement is growing comfort and proficiency within the role of balien. This involves both psychological adjustment and social adaptation.

The Taman do not view the balien's career in terms of professional ambition. Baliens and nonbaliens alike view it as something over which the subject has no control. Nevertheless, limits or barriers to further advancement may be recognized. While some baliens are quick to rise in accomplishment, a few peak at a lower level and indicate no potential for further advancement.

The most striking case is a male balien in his forties who had been initiated in the early 1980s and was, according to his children, an ardent practitioner of bubut therapy. He said he was not fit to become a sarin balien and that he never could become one. He was often called upon to perform the bubut and said that if a balien did not do this as requested, he could become insane. However, he was unable to go any further than this level because of a dream that while he was curing someone in the malai ceremony, his soul traveled to heaven and could not return.

The only case I know of a balien forswearing the profession was a man claiming to be over eighty years old; he had done so because "there was no one to do the weeding." As a result of his lapse of service, he said, his stones disappeared of their own accord. He added that since another male balien in the vicinity had been initiated he did not have to work anymore. Indeed, because of the requirement for male baliens in the menyarung ceremony, it is understandable that he may have been pressed into service long after he would have wanted to retire.

The Efficacy and Social Reality of Balienism

It is useful to differentiate here between reality and efficacy. A sense of reality can derive from nothing more than social consensus, and it is sometimes said that reality itself is a social construction.[5] The question of whether the balien really communicates with the spirit world is one of reality, while the question of whether people really get better because of being treated in a balien ceremony is one of efficacy.[6] During the nearly two years I lived among the Taman, I did not meet or hear of any Taman denying or expressing doubts about the balien's authenticity. This does not mean that all Taman believed that baliens were able to cure the illnesses of their patients.

Taman assert that in certain cases treatment by a balien is necessary, meaning that no other treatment will do and that it satisfactorily resolves the illness. One aspect of effectiveness is the immediacy and directness of the cure. The cures enact instant results: the removal of disease-objects, the return of a missing soul. On being treated by a balien a person is expected to make a quick recovery if the treatment has succeeded.

The first step in being treated by a balien is usually bubut, which in many respects is instrumental. While it is wondrous (thaumaturgical) in that an object is purportedly removed from inside the patient's body merely by rubbing a stone over the skin, the bubut equally involves physical contact between a healer and a patient by way of an instrument—a stone. This is one of the few occasions in all the balien's ceremonies in which there is physical contact between balien and patient. The psychological processes associated with touch may explain much of the therapeutic efficacy of "occult" healing, as Neher (1990: 246) has pointed out. For example, it "can lessen anxiety, promote relaxation, provide distraction, and produce an 'alive' feeling as tactual nerves are stimulated" (Neher 1990: 246).

The balien does not work directly with the patient during the seances; indeed, the patient does not accompany the baliens' convoy when they capture the soul. Such a procedure makes sense given the explanation of illness as resulting from a missing soul that must be located and recaptured. Efforts on the patient's behalf that are witnessed by others contribute to the sense of reality and are congruent with the notions of efficacy in which balienism is grounded.

Ultimately, what deeply impresses people about the reality of balienism are anecdotal reports of the numerous cases of illness that could not be cured by other medication or that had been given up on as hopeless but that improved or seemed to improve after a balien's therapy. A woman recounted the following case:

> My child had all kinds of sicknesses when he was a baby. When I was pregnant with him my stomach was huge, much more than in an average pregnancy. It was difficult to give birth to him. The other ones were easy. A lot of sticky blood came out that was to have been a twin. I dreamed that the child would not get well unless his soul was caught. Otherwise his soul would be taken. I did not believe the dream. My husband and I took the boy to Putussibau for injections even after the doctor had said there was nothing wrong with him. Then the child's eyes were always looking up at the ceiling. I had another dream, this time about my two chickens: one with white feathers, the other with red feathers. Someone came by and said I owed him money and hadn't paid my debt for six years. He said he'd take the red chicken if I didn't pay. I said I did not want to give him the chicken but would pay back the money instead. I felt that the threat of losing the chicken represented the threat of losing my son. After that we called the balien. The boy was eight months old at the time. The balien caught a huge stone. Because of this experience we think he will probably become a balien himself. After that he got better and was never sick again.

In this case the woman became convinced of the appropriateness of a shamanistic cure for her son's illness because of growing dissatisfaction with more conventional medical therapies, and the shock of intrapsychic cues in the form of dreams. One cannot say that the ceremony cathartically cured the baby, but contracting the ceremony assuaged the mother's feelings of helplessness and guilt. The fact that the child recovered fit with the occurrence of the balien's ceremony, and this was recalled as an instance of a life-saving cure by a balien. As far as the villagers were concerned, the child was actually cured by the balien.

In assessing the effectiveness and reality of balien healing one must eventually address the issue of trickery. The skeptic will point out that baliens deliberately trick both the patient and the audience in performing their cures. Does that make them frauds? Robert Barrett (1993) and Clifford Sather (1993) both view trickery as essential to the work of the Iban man-ang—he must trick the spirits. This notion is applicable to the Taman balien, who negotiates with spirits—arguing, begging, singing, dancing, offering food and gifts—but also seeks to outwit them. The spirit steals the patient's soul and the balien steals it back.

Sather has said that the manang "is ideally a trickster."

> The spirits he contends against are believed to work through deception and trickery. Thus they change form at will or employ other subterfuges to cap-ture souls or to injure human victims. To match such adversaries, the *man-ang* must, by necessity, be a master of deception himself. . . . But more than this, those visible actions which the *manang* performs . . . that appear to be "trickery," or sleight of hand, such as producing bits of stone from a patient's head, or wrapping his shoulders in cloth to serve as "wings," may nevertheless have potent effects in the unseen plane in ways that are not immediately perceptible. Just as the shaman's performance during his *pelian* appears to produce "miracles" that defy ordinary comprehension, so the unseen effects of his actions may, in the same way, bring about visible consequences through means that are not directly perceptible to the sens-es, but which are no less "real" all the same. (Sather 1993: 311)

Jane Atkinson (1979: 323) considers the efficacy of the Wana *mabalong* ceremony not in terms of its therapeutic value to the patient but rather in terms of the shaman's self-presentation to the audience. This seems at first to be at most indirectly related to curing effectiveness. But, similar to Barrett's and Sather's interpretations of the Iban manang, Atkinson consid-ers showmanship to be essential. After all, these ceremonies are played out in front of an audience. "A shaman's ability to cure derives from the truth and efficacy of his secret knowledge and associations with spirits. That is, therapeutic effectiveness has its sources in the private side of shamanistic experience—in dealing with hidden realms and beings inaccessible to oth-ers" (Atkinson 1979: 325–326).[7]

> Shamans act out for their audiences a range of feelings familiar to all, but not always publicly acknowledged or admitted in daily life. In this way, they serve as what Lévi-Strauss (1963: 175) has called "professional abre-actors," undergoing and summing up feelings common to all. In doing so, they demonstrate their associations with spirits, who are the sources of shamanistic knowledge and power. It is these associations with spirits which, in the Wana view, are responsible for a shaman's effectiveness in treating patients. (Atkinson 1979: 332)

Baliens themselves commission other baliens to perform these therapies on themselves, paying them the appropriate honoraria, and this seems to demonstrate exquisitely their belief in the reality and efficacy of these cures. A sense of performative efficacy along the lines suggested by Atkinson, Barrett, and Sather must be in operation to explain the coexistence of trickery—a conspiracy of deceit, even—and compliance within the balien system.

Notes

1. Here is one point where the Taman balien departs from Winkelman's characterization of the shaman/healer. But it is possible that Winkelman's generalization stems from errors in the reportage and interpretations of some of his sources, particularly those based on casual observations or the uncorroborated statements of informants. This is a problem inherent in all cross-cultural syntheses, and Winkelman recognizes and attempts to control for it (see Winkelman 1992: 143–172).

2. Baliens may have had high social status in the past. The motif of the rhinoceros hornbill (a less elaborate one than that used by the noble samagat), painted on coffins, trays, walls, and house posts, was a mark of distinction traditionally associated with the pabiring ("middle") rank. According to King, persons of banua ("commoner") traditional social rank were entitled to use this motif of the higher rank if they had proved themselves in war or "acquired prestige as shamans" (King 1985: 91).

3. As described in Chapter 6, objects of customary women's clothing are displayed in the malai ceremony. Their purpose was never explained to me, but it may be surmised that they are associated with Grandmother Siunsun Amas. It is also appropriate to mention here the invocation of a male ancestral practitioner, Grandfather Sanbang, in the Taman practice of divination (see Bernstein 1991: 307–310).

4. Rancour-Laferriere is not referring to an attitude that women are inferior to men or stating that they are subordinated politically and economically. Rather, he is referring specifically to sexuality. This asymmetry is of course adumbrated in customs, rules, symbols, and stereotypes. For example, among the Taman, pekain is paid for a woman's sexual services, and in the event a man has a sexual relationship with a woman to whom he is not married, he must compensate the woman's bilek-family by paying a fine equal to pekain; perabut is viewed as compensation by the man to a woman's bilek-family for taking her away.

5. The definitive statement of this extreme position is that of Berger and Luckmann (1966). See Price-Williams (1987: 252-255) for a pertinent discussion of "the sense of reality," and also Schieffelin (1985).

6. It is also sensible to distinguish between emic and etic interpretations of efficacy, as Etkin (1988) has done.

7. An aspect of Jívaro shamanism described by Harner (1973) provides an interesting counterpoint to the balien's bubut, in which pebbles or other objects are produced in a bowl, signifying the spirits or objects sent by them being extracted from the body. The Jívaro shaman is supposed to suck magical darts from the patient's body, that are then dramatically "vomited" out. Harner was able to learn the shaman's viewpoint on this technique from ex-shamans. In fact the shaman stores the objects in his mouth beforehand, but despite the deception he does not consider this service to be quackery because, unlike his patients, "he knows that the only impor-

tant thing about a *tsentsak* is its supernatural aspect, or essence, which he sincerely believes he has removed from the patient's body" (Harner 1973: 24). The shaman's attitude is one of "pious fraud" (Walsh 1990: 104). He performs this trick primarily for the benefit of the patient, and regards it as essential to the healing process. That is, trickery is used with the deliberate intention of reinforcing the patient's belief in the shaman's healing power, adding to the force of suggestion. Although the Jívaro situation is not fully analogous to that of the Taman, it does indicate the possibility that baliens do not consider their work as sleight-of-hand artists to be deceitful. Such an attitude would bear out Atkinson's point that the essence of shamanism is its performative efficacy rather than its deceitfulness.

8

Conclusion

Anthropologists have discarded the myth that traditional society is somehow unchanging and timeless. Every traditional practice or belief must have either evolved from or succeeded some other form. To conclude this book I want to take a long view of Taman shamanism and traditional healing practices by looking at their changing meanings and purposes in the context of cultural history and evolution. Is it possible to find antecedents to present-day traditions in the absence of documentary records and archeological evidence?

Using colonial administration and church sources, King (1985) has constructed a picture of life in traditional Maloh society (a society that includes the Taman—see Chapter 2). King presents Maloh society as leaving behind its traditional mode of life. The traditional systems of political and social organization King describes were in decline when he studied them. I would argue that the full onslaught of change in the religious and economic spheres has perhaps not been as complete, but the trend of change points in the direction of homogenization and loss of a distinct tradition. As for traditional medicine, it is clear that knowledge of herbal and other medicines from natural products has declined following the availability of manufactured pharmaceutical medicine.

According to King (1985: 50), the Taman have lived in the Upper Kapuas for more than twenty generations. A Taman way of life evolved in the absence of the Indonesian nation, Dutch colonialism, the town of Putussibau, Iban raiders, and the Muslim Malays.[1] The balien's therapies must have been even more important as a form of medicine in the past than they were during the time of my study. It is interesting to speculate about how shamanism may have been organized before the introduction of modern and Malay medicine, when the main alternatives to the balien were traditional herbal and other natural remedies.

In the 1980s the candidate balien had usually sought relief from Malay healers and from doctors and nurses before submitting, out of dissatisfaction and desperation, to the stone-producing ceremonies of the balien. Frequently there was disagreement within the family, usually taking the form of a generation gap: the "conservative" or "traditional" older generation favoring balien treatment and the "modern" younger generation preferring hospitalization. In previous times there would not have been alternative, nonshamanistic explanations of illness or modes of healing. Probably the only choice facing the prospective candidate would have been whether or not to continue toward initiation. Likewise, the choices facing the prospective patient would have been fewer. Balienism would have been part of an all-encompassing way of life different from the plural cultural world in which the Taman now live. The balien system would have provided the only explanation of man's existential condition in illness, suffering, and death, integrated into a living tradition of myth, oratory, and ritual that has now declined. The only other kind of medicine, it may be conjectured, would have been naturalistic herbal medicine, and this may have been integrated with balienism more than is now the case. Remnants of the integration between naturalistic medicine and shamanism can be seen in the balien's own use of medicinal plants, which is based on a presupposition of spirit or object intrusion rather than on a naturalistic notion of medication.

King suggests, plausibly, that following Iban migration to the Upper Kapuas since the mid-nineteenth century, the absorption of Iban into Maloh society led to the assimilation of some Iban folk-medical ideas and vocabulary items (King 1985: 57). Certain of these ideas may be shamanic and in any case would have had an effect on Taman shamanism. Still, the differences between Iban and Taman shamanism are pervasive and immediately apparent (Bernstein 1993a: 177–179). Most fundamentally, the Iban manang is typically male and gifted, while the Taman balien is typically female and afflicted.

The development of shamanism should be seen as an aspect of social and cultural evolution, which is change in the direction of increasing complexity "from a relatively indefinite, incoherent homogeneity to a relatively definite, coherent heterogeneity, through successive differentiations and integrations" (Carneiro 1973: 90). Cultural evolution has taken the form of technological advancement (the increasingly effective harnessing of energy) and increasing social and political complexity. There is clear evidence as well for the evolution of lexical domains and conceptual systems, including color terminology (Berlin and Kay 1969) and the classification of plants and animals (C. Brown 1984).

As a cultural domain, shamanism must also have evolved from a more primitive form. The Taman balien system did not come into being ex nihilo. An approach to the evolution of shamanism is suggested by Winkelman's (1992) distinction between shamans, shaman/healers, mediums, and healers. Winkelman (1992: 58) argues that sedentary residence, agriculture (plant cultivation), and political integration were catalysts promoting the evolution of shamanism.[2] His statistical entailment analysis supports a model of evolution rather than replacement.

As presently constituted, the balien system consists of seven ceremonies, and within these ceremonies five or six distinct procedures carried out by the balien can be ascertained: object extraction, seance (soul travel to contact spirits), spirit conjuring, the capture of spirits and lost souls, and the replacement of lost souls. As for the conceptual models of illness underlying treatment, three or four fundamental ideas are prominent: spirit attack, soul loss or soul capture, and spirit disturbance. The system seems to be comprehensive, and it is impossible to tell from synchronic evidence whether one kind of ceremony or explanation of illness preceded the others. Since the system is also cyclical, tracing its origin seems like a chicken-and-egg proposition. Winkelman's evolutionary model, however, suggests a hypothesis: The true shaman (as opposed to the shaman/healer) is defined by the technique of soul flight. Soul flight is the least-advanced form of shamanism and is associated with the simplest societies. If we accept this hypothesis, seance types of ceremonies such as mangait and especially menindoani would be the most archaic ceremonies. The object extraction technique, bubut, would have been a later development, as would be the concept of illness underlying that treatment: spirit or object intrusion.

The bubut technique is fundamentally different from the other balien techniques. Unlike those essentially shamanic techniques, bubut can be seen as a medical cure of a specific, particular ailment, namely, localized body-part illnesses. It involves both medicines (crushed herbs) and a direct clinical type of encounter with the patient. All the other balien ceremonies only explain the general meaning of illness rather than curing specific illness. Symbolically efficacious though they may be, from the ethnocentric point of view of the outsider, they are not biomedically efficacious. This is most evident in the treatment of the paradoxical illness of the balien-to-be (an illness that seems to presuppose the existence of the system): Catching stones represents the neutralization and materialization of spirits that victimized the patient's soul and sent symptoms of illness. Similarly, the ceremonies locating and contending with spirits and retrieving the patient's soul serve more to explain the illness than to remedy it. It is bubut alone that—all the while employing a spirit-attack model of illness—treats directly the physical symptoms of illness.

The ceremonial capture of spirits as stone marks the balien system as unique, and it is reasonable to suppose that the Taman belien institution evolved independently of other Southeast Asian shamanic traditions. Nevertheless, the basic ingredients of the system are thematic elements in Southeast Asian shamanism. Stones and cordyline leaves, for example, are commonly used in shamanism and other traditional healing in Southeast Asia, though not in the same ways as in the balien system. The hooked tip, though uniquely elaborated as a key feature of shamanism among the

Taman, is a cultural theme in other spheres throughout Borneo.[3] Piercing the eyes and fingertips with hooks is an element of the Iban shaman's initiation, and penis pins are also equated with hooks. The hook motif also appears in classic Bornean iconography. Even more widespread is the word "balien" itself, used (with variations) by many traditional peoples throughout Southeast Asia to refer to healers or magicoreligious practitioners.

The evolution of shamanism did not result in its continual development and refinement but rather in its demise in complex societies, as the role of the shaman was split up and taken over by healers, mediums, priests, sorcerers, diviners, politicians, clowns, and entertainers. While the techniques of magic have remained the same, its value has depreciated. The magician has gone from occupying a sacred role of contacting the spirit world to a profane one of entertainment and amusement. Throughout much of Borneo, shamanism has not only declined but ceased to exist, as societies have embraced (or been embraced by) various processes of modernization. Perhaps it is possible to detect signs of the decline of shamanism among the Taman.

It is possible that the balien system was once more diverse or complex than it was during the time of my study. It is possible, for example, that there were larger concentrations of shamans than there now are and that certain baliens had administrative powers. It is possible that there were two or more kinds of shamans, as is often the case in tribal societies (cf. Crocker 1985; Tsing 1993; Weinstock 1987), and that they had complementary tasks. The density of the symbols, practices, and objects of the balien system suggests that various parts of ceremonies could once have been full ceremonies in themselves. This implies that the present balien system is the simplified remnant of a more complex one. The balien ceremony tabak buse was in decline among the Taman, and as this ceremony appears to be quite different from the other ceremonies, it is possible that it is related to some other ceremonies that are no longer practiced.[4] (Harrisson [1965: 263] mentions an elaboration or perhaps a continuation of this ceremony, *maniang ra buluh ayu dua,* that is no longer practiced.) Indeed, from my interview data and comparisons with the studies of Harrisson and King, I would conclude that Taman ritual and oral tradition as a whole have declined.

The preceding discussion suggests that Taman shamanism may have reached its climax as a cultural institution in the distant past and has been on the wane ever since. While the death of shamanism (and traditional medicine more generally) may be gradual, my impression is that it has usually died because its functions have been replaced by other institutions, especially modern medicine and monotheistic religion.[5] A case in point is the small Kayan community, neighbors of the Taman on the Mendalam River. No traditional medicine of any kind, not even herbalism, was practiced in any of the Kayan villages during the time of my fieldwork. The Kayan had been exposed to Christianity and modern medicine no more than the Taman, yet new baliens were initiated every year in Taman villages, and Taman continually sought the help of baliens in treating illness.

Though the institution of shamanism may have been subject to modifications and even deteriorations over time, it has remained vital. Why? I maintain that becoming and being a balien meets certain important needs rooted in the primary situations of interpersonal relationship: within the family situation and the larger cooperative work groups of which it is a part. Becoming a balien causes a change in status that resolves those problems, enabling a person to function normally and escape from illness.

Illness is not only interpreted through a cultural knowledge system but can be used (though it may not be) to express resistance or dissatisfaction with one's role or position. Nancy Scheper-Hughes (1994) has suggested that the body can be used *subversively* to protest and complain through illness and modalities such as spirit possession. Illness, according to Scheper-Hughes (1994: 232), can express anger, fear, resentment, or envy. It can represent an act of refusal—"a refusal to work, a refusal to endure, a refusal to 'cope'" (Scheper-Hughes 1994: 238). In the case of the Taman, I would conclude that the various components making up the balien's predisposing illness—dissociation, depression, delusion, and somatization—express problems of adaptation within the family situation, including gender and sexuality. The balien system not only *normalizes* such an expression of complaint through a recognized process of initiation but *resolves* the problem in a way that gives those afflicted who undergo the full process a socially valid role and inverts their position from that of patient to healer.

It is difficult to know whether the transformation to balien status was always wrapped up in conflict about the domestic situation and family issues as opposed to other problems of identity. Was balienism ever associated more closely with the main forms of power? Could being a balien have been a route to power or social influence among the Taman? King's research suggests the possibility that baliens previously enjoyed exalted status. Propitiatory or piacular ceremonies outside the realm of healing are performed by baliens among the Embaloh (King 1985: 194). Persons who have distinguished themselves through meritorious acts—and this includes baliens—are entitled to larger food offerings at their funerals than others (King 1985: 92).[6]

The hereditary rank system was the main basis of power and epitomized the concept of value in archaic Taman society (see Chapter 2). King's materials at the very least suggest that balien status was culturally valued to the extent that it entitled baliens to override low ascribed rank and enjoy the privileges of high rank. Judging from King's data, it was mainly women who advanced themselves this way. Female baliens of banua rank, like male warriors of that rank, were entitled to use decorative motifs associated with the higher pabiring rank (King 1985: 91). Unlike most people of banua rank, a few could trace lengthy genealogies because they had prominent ancestors:

"big men," mantri ("aristocrat's right-hand man"), and baliens (King 1985: 132). Men's claims on symbols of honor (and implicitly virtue) rise in proportion to their achievements in the quintessentially masculine pursuits of warfare and headhunting. The only route to such honor open to women is that of the balien.

There is no evidence to suggest that Taman baliens were ever different from what they are now, in that they are selected on the basis of otherwise incurable illness and are predominantly female.[7] The cross-cultural work of Winkelman (1992: 45) validates for magicoreligious practitioners the truism that power and socioeconomic position are correlated with male domination. Although Winkelman has not quantified this correlation, the idea that a female-dominated profession could serve not only as healers but as the priesthood for the main system of belief and ritual and could control the main symbols of power within the society goes against the findings not only of Winkelman's survey but also Lewis's (1971). Baliens' work as healers is indeed highly valued by the Taman. Their miraculous cures are marveled at, and great baliens of yore are commemorated. But King's findings on the high status of baliens *outside the domain of healing* are not corroborated by my studies, and it is difficult to interpret their meaning in understanding the status and organization of shamanism in archaic Taman society.

Following Winkelman's hypothesis of the social transformation of the shaman, shamanism would have predated the rank system among the Taman. King's historical evidence suggests that the status of baliens remained high during the florescence of the rank system. No explicit mention of the rank system was made in any balien ceremonies I studied. The closest implicit reference to it is in the use of the sulekale, a figurine offered to spirits in exchange for the patient's soul with the words, "Take this as your slave."[8] While the kalangkang used in the menyarung ceremony is decorated with traditional motifs (Harrisson 1966), these are not taken to be "symbols of social differentiation" (Whittier 1973).

If the forerunners of contemporary baliens had broad ritual powers extending beyond healing, as King's study implies, it is possible that their rituals and the cosmological knowledge underpinning them related to and perhaps legitimized the rank system. In an age when resources were controlled by the samagat nobility, persons of lesser rank may have been restricted in gaining admission to the association—and a cure of their illness—through initiation. Baliens may have worked hand in hand with the samagat as gatekeepers. Admission would have been a sign of endorsement of the ancestress and might have been taken to mean individual inspiration.

These speculations about how balien ideologies arose and how they were previously constituted stem from a reading of Roger Keesing's (1987) critique of symbolic and interpretive anthropology. According to Keesing, symbolic and interpretive anthropologists consider systems of belief and knowledge (e.g., ritual knowledge) only in terms of meaning.[9] The results of purely symbolic analysis could lead to bias, giving precedence to elitist interpretations. Besides creating "webs of significance" (the symbolic anthropologist's object of study), systems of belief and knowledge constitute ideologies serving the interests of those who control and produce that knowledge. Ritual knowledge is produced, controlled, maintained, and distributed. What or whose interests, Keesing asks, are served by the maintenance of these systems of knowledge? This question may be asked about the balien system. While balienism consists of public performances, the knowledge system behind those performances, the mysteries and secrets of balienism, are decidedly not open to the public.

Baliens not only use mystification but interpret the unseen realm (including the land of the dead and the journey to it) for the society. As Eliade (1964: 509) has written, it is probable that "many features of 'funerary geography,' as well as some themes of the mythology of death, are the result of the ecstatic experiences of shamans." Primordial baliens—perhaps including the real-life Grandmother Siunsun Amas herself—were charismatic figures, inspired classic shamans rather than practitioners of routinized healing activities.[10] Present-day baliens, however, are not charismatic. Unlike the Meratus Dayak shaman Uma Adang, whose mysterious personality, and eccentric and riveting performance style, are described vividly by Tsing (1987), the Taman shamans described here and are not creative manipulators of symbols. They would not be outstanding theatrical performers, and they could not be likened to prophets or saviors. While some people may have disbelieved in the baliens' healing methods, as they do to this day, the successful cures worked by the baliens would have sustained and served to legitimize the system. It is here that the fact that those cured at the highest level of the system become members of the group becomes significant.

Baliens are "created" by being formally inducted into a group; they practice as members of the group; and their doctrine or code is completely group based. (The only signs of individual variation seem to be in the names given to some of the stones, which are revealed in dreams, and in some of the specific details of bubut technique.) Their ideology is a comprehensive system, not one that can be filled in or added to. There is little room for creative manipulation of symbols or innovation, unlike the Malay dukuns described in Chapter 3, who do not undergo initiation but may enter their healing specialty through any of a number of routes. Compared with baliens, dukuns are specific in differentiating between the various illnesses and curing them. Their knowledge can be added to in a piecemeal fashion, and innovation and eclecticism are permissible. They may also impart any or all of their knowledge to others as they see fit; those who acquire some of this knowledge are not required to undergo a life-transforming initiation ritual.

In answer to Keesing's question of who benefits, it is the baliens themselves who benefit, by maintaining secrecy, although they benefited more in the past than they do now. But Keesing's implicit Marxism must be confronted head-on: The baliens' interests never represented class interests. Balienism is open to all afflicted and contains no elements of an ideology of social differentiation. (Even if the balien could in effect be bumped up a notch in the rank hierarchy, as King's data suggest, this benefit did not radiate to the balien's family members or offspring.) On the other hand, there are no signs that the balien system protests the inequities of the rank system or patriarchy. While King's findings about Embaloh shamanism are intriguing, on the balance, the Taman balien system does not significantly entail rules, symbols, or representations of social hierarchy.

It is now clear that shamanism has outlived the "traditional" social system based on rank as well as the "traditional system" of political leadership, both of which are aspects of Taman adat. (When I inquired about why no one had stepped forward to succeed the Sibau temenggung after he died, I was told that no one possessed sufficient understanding of the adat to fill the position.) Why have not the numerous and interrelated factors that led to the decline of the systems of rank and leadership—economics, colonial administration, education, monotheistic religion, and nationalism/independence/Pancasila—also caused the downfall of the balien system? For the answer to this question, we should consider the part of the rank system that *has* endured: marriage payments and associated fines. The customs pertaining to the *domestic sphere* have been maintained and even updated (required sums in cash transactions rising periodically with inflation). The balien domain—the treatment of illness—falls entirely within the domestic sphere. The illness complexes leading to initiation seem also to arise from situations in domestic life and perhaps socialization. Although the balien's illness is a response to these problems that cannot be resolved directly, it is not a calculated, rational means to an end.

Spirit neutralization and initiation are mechanisms for Taman, especially women, to deal with needs arising from sexual impulses. According to Neher (1990: 112ff.), sexual *repression* is commonly a factor underlying mystical experience: The fact that sexual imagery is described in visions Neher takes as evidence that the repression is incomplete. The kinds of fantasy related to the balien's illness are the results of specific forms of repression of the pleasure principle. Various forms of "surplus repression" may arise as the result of particular cultural emphases in the expression of the reality principle (Obeyesekere 1981: 165–167). No mechanism or institution within Taman society has either eliminated the need addressed by initiation or vanquished the initiation process. Those who face irremediable problems, whether or not they are somatic, and have tried all other kinds of remedies may seek refuge in the treatment of the balien. Balien therapy may not treat the disease itself (unlike the doctor's medicine), but it may remedy the sick person's general sense of unwellness and incapacity to function. For those whose somaticized problems are related to coping, the solution to their problems may lie in becoming a balien. It may continue to do so for a long time to come. The persistence of the Taman balien system may be added to the record of ethnographic evidence that the world has not seen the last of "traditional" shamanism.

Notes

1. The Taman way of life did not evolve in isolation. According to oral tradition, King (1985: 52) writes, "forest people" such as the Punan, Bukat, and Bukitan already lived in the Upper Kapuas at the time of the arrival of the Maloh. While the major influxes of Chinese, Iban, Kayan, and Malay to the Upper Kapuas came in the early nineteenth century, it seems likely that the Taman had at least some relations with those groups before that time; and there must have been other peoples in contact with the Taman. Relations with the Iban have been close and to an unusual extent friendly (Harrisson 1965: 246) whereas relations with the Chinese would have been based on mutually rewarding commercial interests. But other Dayak groups, especially the Kayan and Kantuk, were dreaded enemies of the Taman.

2. Winkelman does not distinguish between agriculture and horticulture, that is, shifting cultivation.

3. Harrisson (1965: 322) mentions that the fishing hook is viewed as a means of "hooking down" the spirit world and writes, "As such it plays a vital role—often in natural, accidental, stone or deer's antler 'hooks'—especially in Kayan and Kenyah *shamanism*. It is not such a deep idea with the Iban, however."

4. My data indicate that this ceremony serves no function that is not served by any other ceremony. This may have contributed to its obsolescence.

5. Religious ideology, and those disseminating or enforcing it, not only may have replaced shamanistic ideology by satisfying or obviating the needs it met but may have stamped it out or suppressed it as heresy.

6. The logic behind this privilege is that the menyarung ceremony is considered an important feast (gawa').

7. Chu (1978: 192–195), following certain early writers on Iban shamanism, speculates that the institution of the *manang bali,* the transformed (i.e. transvestite) shaman, is evidence that shamanism was originally a female role among the Iban, and that the manang is ideally a woman. According to one legend cited by Chu, "Grandmother Ini, the only sister in the ancestral Iban family, is recognized as the first and greatest of all shaman-doctors" (Chu 1978: 194). See also S. Murray 1992, and compare Winzeler 1993. The classic statement on the Iban manang is that of Derek Freeman (1967).

8. The concept of the slave also transferred to customary law, in that certain amounts of money were paid that formerly would have been transacted in slaves.

9. For present purposes, symbolic and interpretive anthropology are synonymous. See also Dolgin et al. 1977; Marcus and Fischer 1986; Rabinow and Sullivan 1979.

10. Lewis seems to have in mind this classic model of shamanism rather than a shaman/healer model, which comes closer to the nature of the Taman balien, when he characterizes the shaman as "an inspired prophet and healer, a charismatic religious figure" (Lewis 1986: 88). But Grim's distinction between the shaman and the prophet shows why baliens are not prophets. Unlike the prophet, the shaman "does not develop a vision of historical destiny. . . . There is no abiding covenant between the tribe and the spirits that shamans promote in the pursuit of their religious vocation" (Grim 1983: 185).

Appendix A:

Glossary

This is a glossary of Taman and other words relevant to this book. The reader is referred to Diposiswoyo 1985, Hudson 1970, King 1976b, and King 1985 for more complete word lists. Language in parentheses following a term indicates that the term is not a Taman word. However, many Taman words are also accepted in other languages and in some cases borrowed from them.

Adat. Custom, customary law.

Angin (Malay). Wind.

Ansan. Fleck, speck, tiny pebble.

Antu. Ghost.

Antumelet. Herpes.

Apais. Ill, sick.

Apuan. Shortness of breath, bronchial asthma, or other upper respiratory tract illness.

Badet. See **Najam.**

Badi (Malay). Revenge in the form of illness from a spirit for harming or violating it.

Badi api. Fire badi.

Badi kucing (alt. **badi pusa'**). Cat badi.

Badi lumantik (alt. **badi semadak**). Black-ant badi.

Badi turos (alt. **badi pancak**). Stake badi.

Bajoak. Gastroenteritis.

Baju kalawat. Blouse worn by the balien when performing ceremonies.

Bala buloh. Bundle of sixty twigs used as an offering to the balien goddess **Piang Siunsun Amas** in **menindoani, mengadengi,** and **menyarung** ceremonies. Made out of bamboo in **menindoani** ceremony and out of **tabas pusa'** (Clerodendrum) for use in the other ceremonies. Literal translation: Split bamboo.

Balasan. Revenge. For example, **dabalas jalu,** revenge by a being.

Balien. Shaman.

Balien baba. Male shaman. The **menyarung** ceremony requires that at least one male shaman participate.

Balien bibinge. Female shaman.

Balien sarin. Master shaman.

Bangkar. Illness, fever, the beginning (mild) stage of disease.

Banua. (1) Village unit. (2) Commoner rank.

Batu Balien. Stone from **sai** used as part of the balien's equipment to cure disease.

Batu Kait. Stone used in **mangait** ceremony.

Batu Karangan. Ordinary stone.

Baungau. Insane.

Belang. Leprosy.

Bilek (Iban). Longhouse apartment. (Taman: **tindo'an.**) **Bilek**-family. Family unit, usually multigenerational, inhabiting one longhouse apartment.

Bua'. Minimum unit for calculating fines in legal cases.

Bubut. Balien cure in which a stone (**Batu Balien**) dipped in a medicinal herb is stroked over a body part to remove from the body a spirit being or projectile object delivered by a spirit.

Bukit Tilung. Mountain in Mandai Subdistrict, final resting place of the dead.

Buling. Period of ritual prohibition following burial of a dead person.

Buluh ayu. Decorated bamboo pole with split end used in **menyarung** ceremony to achieve contact with spirit world; held up while chanting.

Buluh merindu. "Longing bamboo." Magical reed said to grow naturally at **Bukit Tilung.** Well known as main ingredient in **jayau.**

Cocok. Fitting, appropriate.

Dabalas jalu. See **Badi** and **Balasan**.

Dawawa jalu. "Captured/taken away by a being." Affliction of candidate baliens, including hysterical symptoms.

Dugal (Upper Kapuas Malay). Stomach cramps, gastritis, said to be caused by a disorder of circulation resulting from the entrance of hot wind into the body.

Dukun (Malay). Wizard, folk healer. While the term is used in this text to refer to Malay healers, it can encompass the balien as well.

Dung suri (Iban: **sabang**). Leaf of the *Cordyline fructicosa* plant used in balien ceremonies especially to catch spirits. **Dung** means "leaf."

Ilmu gaib. Magic.

Ilmu (Malay). Mystical knowledge, magic.

Ilmu sihir. Witchcraft.

Jalu. Object, in the context of illness, a spirit being.

Jalu tio. Measles caused by spirits.

Jang. Poison.

Jayau. Love medicine.

Jengkal. Palm's breadth, or the distance between the thumb and second finger when spread apart.

Jimat (alt. **zimat, azimat**). Amulet.

Jin. Goblin, spirit monster.

Juaran. A medicinal leaf prominent in Malay medicine.

Kait. Hook. See **mangait, pangait.**

Kalangkang. Tray containing offerings suspended to form a sort of hut, which is at the center of the menyarung ceremony and in which the initiate sits when not dancing.

Kalo'an. Miscarriage. (From **alo'**, "fall.")

Kalong. Throat.

Kapaisan. Disease, illness.

Karangan. Sudden sickness, fainting.

Karawan. A grave illness, the symptoms of which include dementia.

Karimut (alt. **kerumut, gerumut**). (1) Measles. (2) Traditional girdle made of small silver rings, a well-known part of traditional Taman craftsmanship. The **karimut** is placed with other traditional finery to attract the spirits.

Kempunan (alt. **kaponan**). Revenge by a spirit or ghost for omitting to carry out or complete an intended or expected action.

Ketika. Augur.

Kombong. Meeting.

Kulombo'. A braided cube made of leaves and filled with rice, used in propitiatory ceremonies.

Kunti (alt. **munti, punti**). Protective charm causing severe illness to anyone who violates it.

Laso (alt. **paren**). Penis.

Lingkutut. Knee.

Maag (Indonesian, orig. Dutch). Gastritis, gastric or duodenal ulcer.

Malai. Balien performance to catch the soul.

Maloh (poss. alt. **banuaka'**). Aggregate term referring to the Taman, Kalis, and Embaloh ethnic groups.

Manang (Iban). Shaman. (This term has entered the Taman language such that it is interchangeable with the Taman word **balien.** For analytic purposes, I use the term here to refer to Iban shamans only, except in direct quotes from informants.)

Mangait. Balien ceremony to locate and call back the soul.

Maniang. To heal, particularly as applied to baliens.

Maniang aso. A healing seance (**mangait**) performed, unusually, during the daytime.

Manidu'. Phase of the **malai** ceremony in which two baliens work together with one **pangait** to locate the patient's soul.

Marem. Palm wine, used in all ceremonial occasions.

Melepos. Ceremonially accepting food or drink to avoid exposing oneself to **kempunan.**

Mengadengi. Exorcism ceremony in which a stone is caught.

Menindoani. Advanced balien seance to locate, capture, and bring back the soul from heaven.

Menyarung. Balien's initiation ceremony lasting three days and nights.

Mintuari. Person, body.

Mipiki. A ceremony in which a chicken is waved to brush away a bad dream.

Mok. A mug. As a unit of measure, a mugful, or about 8 ounces.

Mui ajau. Bad dream. Cause of bad luck.

Munusi. The magical withdrawal of a pathological splinter from deep within the body.

Najam. Gastric or respiratory pains in the chest attributed to assaults by spirits.

Nunuk (alt. **kayu ara**). Strangling fig/banyan trees (*Ficus* spp.), thought to be repositories of spirits.

Pabiring. Middle rank.

Pais. Pain, disease.

Pais layu-layu. "Pining-away illness."

Pamari'an. See **sai**.

Pancasila. A doctrine underlying the Indonesian constitution of 1945, and consisting of five axioms: belief in one God, humanity that is just and civilized, national unity, democracy guided by representative deliberation, and social justice for all Indonesians.

Pangait. Hook-tipped pole used by the balien in a number of ceremonies.

Pangkam (alt. **kelitau**). Slave.

Parangka'. Back, spine.

Pekain. Payment given to the bride's family from the groom's family at the time of marriage and returned in case of divorce. Twice the **pekain** for brides of **banua** or **pabiring** rank is paid for marriage to a woman of **samagat** rank. The value of **pekain** is traditionally calculated in gongs or finery, but a monetary equivalent is now accepted.

Piang Siunsun Amas. Goddess of the baliens. (**Piang** means "grandmother.")

Polek. Medicine.

Puskesmas (Pusat Kesehatan Masyarakat). Public Health Center, clinic.

Rabe. Metal hook inserted into fingertips and used to pierce outer layer of eyeball in **menyarung** ceremony.

Rematik. Rheumatism.

Sabang. See **Dung suri.**

Sai (alt. **pamari'an**). Spirit or demon, thought to cause disease.

Sakang. Poison or antidote.

Sakule'. "Like that," appropriate, fitting.

Samagat. Noble rank.

Sampi. Incantation.

Sangka' (alt. **sangga**). Antidote.

Sarung ase. "Rice hat." Large sun hat from which rice panicles and various kinds of leaves and fishes are suspended around the edge, worn in the **menyarung** ceremony.

Saur. Shrub, the succulent leaves of which are used by the balien in bubut therapy.

Sekitam (Malay). "Black sickness," leading to **karawan.**

Sengkalan. A small fine for minor offenses within customary law.

Singko. Deformed, handicapped.

Sulekale. Sugar cane carved into replica of a person, offered by a balien.

Sumangat. Soul.

Sumangat dualapan. Soul-of-eight. The duality and multiplicity of the souls in Taman belief.

Suri. See **dung suri.**

Tabak buse. Seance and chant similar to **menindoani,** but uses drums instead of other balien equipment.

Taengen. Woven rattan basket, can be used to contain balien's stones.

Tamang. Double. A stone that is a double or replica of a person, in a mystical sense.

Tamatoa. Parent or elder.

Tampun. A pebble removed from the patient's head in the **bubut** therapy, considered dangerous.

Tantamu (Malay: **mentemu**). Yellow ginger, a rhizome used in Taman and Malay medicine.

Tanung. Oracle.

Tapu'. Fontanel. (Place from which the soul enters and exits the body.)

Tauning. The balien's beaded bracelet, strung with cast-iron bells.

Tepas. Malay therapy in which disease is magically removed from the patient's body and brushed off.

Tikolo'. Headdress beaded with coconut cubes and worn by balien in the **men-yarung** ceremony.

Timang. Chant, epic, or saga.

Tolang. Bone(s).

Ulu. Head.

Ulu ati. Liver.

Wase. (1) Adze. (2) (alt. **penyalak, kangkuang basi**). Metal instrument resembling an awl or small adze head used by the balien during the **malai** ceremony by striking it against a sword blade to produce a ringing sound.

Yang Suka. God, or a judge at **Bukit Tilung.**

Appendix B:

Key to Plants Used in Medicine and Ritual

Local name	Family	Name	Uses
Abung-abung	Asteraceae	*Blumea balsamifera* (L.) D.C.	Boiled in water and drunk to treat shivers, headaches, and labor pains.
Banoh	Acanthaceae	*Gendarussa vulgaris* Nees.	Requirement for kalangkang.
Bararan kuning	Menispermaceae	*Fibraurea chloroleuca* Miers.	Vines are boiled and water drunk to treat hepatitis.
Bararan sasait	Rubiaceae	*Uncaria sclerophylla* (Hunter) Roxb.	Water boiled and either drunk as tea or put on nipple of nursing mother to treat stomachaches and thrush in children.
Bunga balien	Lycopodiaceae	*Lycopodium phlegmaria* L.	Requirement for kalangkang.
Bunga endong	Apiaceae	*Centella asiatica* (L.) Urb.	Boiled as tea and drunk to reduce swelling.
Bunga randi'	Malvaceae	*Hibiscus rosa-sinensis* L.	Leaves are crushed and compressed on infected wounds to draw out pus.
Bungkang	Myrtaceae	*Syzigium polyanthum* (Wight.) Walp.	Bark is used in treating diarrhea.

179

Cangkok	Euphorbiaceae	*Sauropus androgynus* (L.) Merr.	Reduces body heat in fever, or mixed with chili pepper leaves, yeast, and hot water to induce labor in women.
Dung ilung	Araceae	*Homalomena propiqua* Schott.	Burned to frighten ghosts.
Dung kalangkang	Ophioglossaceae	*Helminostachys zeylanica* (L.) Hook	Boiled as tea to cure internal illnesses, especially of the liver.
Dung malu	Fabaceae	*Mimosa pudica* L.	Ashes of the burnt leaves heal wounds.
Juaran	Rubiaceae		Crushed in water and rubbed on the body to treat infection, swelling, and fever.
Kalambibit	Convolvulacea	*Merremia umbellata* (L.) Hall.f.	Eaten by baliens in menyarung ceremony.
Karambai	Rubiaceae	*Psychotria* sp.	Boiled in water, which is brushed on the skin to treat scabies.
Kulat tembus	Polyporaceae	*Amaurodermia* sp.	Burned, mixed with water, and brushed on limbs that have fallen asleep.
Kumis kucing	Labiatae	*Orthosiphon stamieus* Benth.	Drunk as tea to treat urinary tract disorders.
Limpa dutana	Scrophulariaceae	*Lindernia viscosa* (Hornem) Merr.	Whole plant boiled and water drunk as medicine for respiratory ailments and malaria.
Lukai	Annonaceae		Bark and leaves are burned to frighten ghosts, especially in cases of stomachaches. The ashes are rubbed on the abdomen.
Melor	Fabaceae	*Cassia surattensis* Burm.f.	Ritual use by balien; treats fever.

Memali	Leeaceae	*Leea indica* (Burm.f.) Merr.	Crushed leaves absorb pus.
Mematekan	Verbenaceae	*Callicarpa longifolia* Lamk.	To treat malaria, shivers, or labor pains.
Olong-olong	Nepenthaceae	*Nepenthes bicalcarata* Hk.f.	Boiled and drunk as tea to treat dysentery.
Patalo'	Loranthaceae	*Dendrophthora pentandra* (L.) Miq.	Burned and dropped into dental caries; said to eat worms that are parasitic of the teeth.
Rambean	Euphorbiaceae	*Baccaurea motleyana* M.A.	The bark is boiled and the water is put into the eyes.
Riribu	Schizaeaceae	*Lygodium flexuosum* (L.) Sw.	Requirement for kalangkang; boiled for tea to treat nervous and muscular tension.
Saur	Zingiberaceae	*Kaempferia galanga* L.	Used by balien to remove spirits from the body, especially in children.
Serai	Poaceae	*Cymbopogon nardus* (L.) Rendle	For hoarse throat, the plant is boiled and drunk as tea.
Serunggan	Fabaceae	*Cassia alata* (L.) Ridley	Crushed on skin to treat fungal itch and ringworm, or boiled as tea to treat stomach cramps.
Suri	Liliaceae	*Cordyline fruticosa* (L.) Backer	Used in catching spirits; has some other medicinal uses.
Tabas pusa'	Verbenaceae	*Clerodendrum* cf. *squamatum* Vahl.	Requirement for kalangkang.
Tanpasui	Zingiberaceae		Requirement for kalangkang.
Tantamu	Zingiberaceae	*Curcuma xanthorrhiza* (L.) Roxb.	Rubbed on body to remove spirits; also drunk as an elixir.

Tapang uran	Euphorbiaceae	*Pedilanthus tithymaloides* (L.) Poit	Sap used to treat bites from snakes, scorpions, and centipedes.
Taraksio	Rutaceae	*Tetractomia obovata* Merr.	Requirement for kalangkang.
Tarangga'	Balsaminaceae	*Impatiens cf. balsamina* L.	Leaves are burnt and ashes rubbed on the body to guard against infection.
Tentabong	Melastomaceae	*Medinilla* sp.	Requirement for kalangkang.

Appendix C:

Field Methods

I first contacted the Taman in September 1984 and conducted research among them from December 1985 to May 1986, August 1986 to January 1987, and August 1987 to January 1988. I first studied a Taman village located on the Kapuas River, devoting most of my effort to language and vocabulary. I soon changed my focus to the Sibau Taman, however. Most of the cases described in this book occurred in Sibau Hilir, the largest Taman village (its population was 1,057 in 1987). However, in the course of my studies, I collected data on illness and traditional medicine in every Taman village except Eko Tambai. (This village, located on the Kapuas River between Melapi and Siut, was unusual in that living among the villagers were two U.S. missionaries and their families.) I also conducted research in the nearby Malay town of Putussibau and adjacent hamlets. I began my research using the Indonesian language, but I made an effort to learn Taman (*kada banuaka'*), and eventually I was able to converse in this language and understand the conversations of others.

I strove to include in my study people representing a large range of village society. My prime informants included men, women, and children; elderly and young; headmen, shop owners, hunters, and common farmers; high school graduates and people who had never been to school.

I collected from each interview subject general data about household and kinship. Through the study of family life, I identified cases of illness and curing. By studying these cases and interviewing folk healers as well as patients and their families, I developed vocabulary lists about illness and medicine. With improved understanding of Taman culture gained through participant observation, I was able to develop a set of questions to elicit concepts about the causes, cures, and associations of the various diseases. These questions were put to a range of informants. In a similar manner I also questioned informants about kinds of medicines and the different spirits. (With the help of informants, I developed interview protocols in Taman.) The purpose of these questions was to discover the conceptual basis of Taman ethnomedicine, the content of medical knowledge, and the distribution and variation of this knowledge within the village community.

Besides formal and prearranged interviews, I also had many informal and spontaneous interviews with informants. Over time I became involved with village activities and developed close relationships with many villagers that extended beyond the research. Information from casual conversations and interactions contributed to my understanding of Taman society to a great extent.

I studied numerous cases of cures by folk healers, recording the events on tape whenever possible and interviewing concerned parties. Whenever I learned of a case of illness or a healing event, I tried to visit the house of the concerned party and requested permission to record the event. The performances were public and I was never denied access, although I was occasionally asked not to take photographs.

With the possible exception of this photographic intrusion, my presence did not affect the behavior of any of the participants. With all my equipment, I felt conspicuous, though I tried to be as unobtrusive as possible. Knowing of the baliens' proclivity for cigarettes in certain ceremonies, I tried to remember to bring some along for them, but I never made any other contributions toward any healing ceremonies.

Tape-recorded ceremonies were later transcribed and translated with the help of informants. I also interviewed my informants about past illnesses within their families. My methodological concern was to collect data from the perspectives associated with the various roles in healing events. For example, by interviewing the patient and his or her family, I learned about the history of the illness and the attempts to cure it. In time, the healers became familiar with me and regarded my presence as commonplace, if not always welcome.

Some U.S. anthropologists feel that the word "informant," referring to any person whose interview statements provide data used in constructing ethnographic texts, is outmoded, patronizing, and easily misunderstood to mean "informer" and, by extension, "traitor." Calling these people "consultants" instead of "informants" would perhaps give a sense of equal partnership and collaboration. It is also possible to substitute for "informant" words like "friend" or "acquaintance," in recognition of the fact that ethnography is rarely a formal process. While I am now cognizant of these problems surrounding the word "informant," they were far from my mind when I conducted my fieldwork. Some of my informants were my friends, and others were not, but I thought of them all as informants: I tried not to let personal feelings get in the way when I was interviewing or observing a person.

I made it clear at the outset that I was collecting data on Taman culture and especially traditional medicine for my thesis and that I hoped to write a book on the subject. I had letters showing that I was a student affiliated with Gadjah Mada University and a signed statement indicating that I complied with the guidelines of Indonesian Institute of Sciences for conducting research. I explained that I would regret writing anything inaccurate and that I needed to have correct information in order to produce a reliable account of Taman culture and medicine. I asked people if they would agree to be my informants and whether I could quote information from them in my work. I said that I would not publish anyone's real name. I interviewed informants in their free time, though at times I also accompanied them when they were working. I did not pay people for interviews, but I did give gifts and do favors for the many people who aided me in conducting the research. Not all of the people quoted or described in this book were informants, in the sense that they were not interviewed by me.

Appendix D:

Note on the Value of the Rupiah

The value of the Indonesian rupiah at the time of this study can be elucidated by stating the rate of exchange against the U.S. dollar and by giving the prices of typical consumer items. At the time my fieldwork began in late 1985, U.S. $1.00 was the equivalent of about Rp 1,120; or, put another way, Rp 1,000 was equal to U.S. $0.89. The following year the economy fluctuated throughout the world, and on September 12, 1986, the rupiah was devalued to an exchange rate of Rp 1,644 to U.S. $1.00 or U.S. $0.60 to Rp 1,000. However, the prices of consumer goods were little affected.

In late 1985, the price of rice in the Putussibau market was Rp 600 per kilogram; packets of instant noodle soup (Indomie) were Rp 150 each; and sugar cost Rp 800 per kilogram. Coffee cost Rp 5,000 per kilogram; sweetened condensed milk cost Rp 700 per small can; and sardines cost Rp 300 per small can. Kerosene cost Rp 375 per kilogram. Live chickens cost Rp 2,500–3,000 per kilogram. Pork cost Rp 1,000–1,500 per kilogram, and dried fish cost Rp 2,000 per kilogram. Cigarettes had an average price of Rp 400–600 per pack.

During the time of my study, the price of processed rubber (a major source of income for the Taman) reached and surpassed Rp 1,000 per kilogram. At a shop in a small village in 1986, rice was purchased for Rp 800–900 per gantang ("gallon," or 4.04 liters, weighing 2.5 kilograms) at the conclusion of the harvest in April. In November of that year, the same shopkeeper paid Rp 1,100 per gantang of rice and sold it for Rp 1,200.

Appendix E:

Musical Description of the Balien Chant

The balien's chant includes a verse sung by the leader, followed by a chorus sung by all the other participating baliens, consisting of the final few syllables of the verse. The melody of the chorus is as follows:

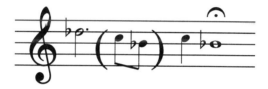

The tune in which the verse is sung uses a free-style permutation of the same notes that are used in the chorus.

Bibliography

Abse, D. Wilfred. 1959. "Hysteria." In *American Handbook of Psychiatry,* edited by Silvano Arieti, vol. 1, pp. 272–292. New York: Basic Books.

Adelaar, K. Alexander. 1994. "The classification of the Tamanic languages." In *Language Contact and Change in the Austronesian World,* edited by Tom Dutton and Darrel T. Tryon, pp. 1–42. Berlin: Mouton de Gruyter.

Ali As, M. 1967. "Perdata Adat Perzinahan Ditindjau Dari Adat—Agama— Pantjasila" ("Customary Civil Law Concerning Adultery, as Approached from Adat, Religion, and Pancasila"). Skripsi Sardjana Hukum, Universitas Negeri Tandjungpura.

Anyang, Y. C. Thambun. 1985. "Hukum Adat Perkawinan Daya Taman di Kecamatan Putussibau" ("Taman Dayak marriage customs in the Putussiban Subdistrict"). Penataran Ilmu Pengetahuan Hukum Adat Pada Fakultas Hukum, Universitas Syiah Kuala Darussalam, Banda Aceh.

Appell, G. N., editor. 1976. *The Societies of Borneo: Explorations in the Theory of Cognatic Social Structure.* Special Publication of the American Anthropological Association, no. 6. Washington, DC: American Anthropological Association.

Atkinson, Jane Monnig. 1979. "Paths of the Spirit Familiars: A Study of Wana Shamanism." Ph.D. dissertation, Stanford University.

———. 1987a. "The effectiveness of shamans in an Indonesian ritual." *American Anthropologist* 89: 342–355.

———. 1989. *The Art and Politics of Wana Shamanship.* Berkeley: University of California Press.

———. 1992. "Shamanisms today." *Annual Review of Anthropology* 21: 307–330.

Balunus, H. M. Baroamas Jabang. n.d. "Asal Mula Kejadian Dunia dan Manusia." ("The Genisis of the World and Mankind"). Unpublished manuscript.

Barrett, Robert J. 1993. "Performance, effectiveness, and the Iban manang." In *The Seen and the Unseen: Shamanism, Mediumship and Possession in Borneo,* edited by Robert L. Winzeler, pp. 235–279. Borneo Research Council Monograph Series, vol. 2. Williamsburg, VA: Borneo Research Council.

Baudrillard, Jean. 1981 [1972]. *For a Critique of the Political Economy of the Sign,* translated and with an introduction by Charles Levin. St. Louis, MO: Telos Press.

Beidelman, T. O. 1993. *Moral Imagination in Kaguru Modes of Thought.* Washington, D.C.: Smithsonian Institution Press.Bell, Catherine. 1992. *Ritual Theory, Ritual Practice.* New York: Oxford University Press.

Bell, Catherine. 1992. *Ritual Theory, Ritual Practice.* New York: Oxford University Press.

Berger, Peter L., and Thomas Luckmann. 1966. *The Social Construction of Reality: A Treatise in the Sociology of Knowledge.* New York: Doubleday.

Berlin, Brent, and Paul Kay. 1969. *Basic Color Terms: Their Universality and Evolution.* Berkeley: University of California Press.

Bernstein, Jay H. 1990. "The infusion of teachers from Eastern Indonesia into West Kalimantan." In *Patterns of Migration in Southeast Asia,* edited by Robert R. Reed, pp. 182–190. Occasional Paper no. 16. Berkeley: Centers for South and Southeast Asian Studies, University of California, Berkeley.

————. 1991. "Taman Ethnomedicine: The Social Organization of Sickness and Medical Knowledge in the Upper Kapuas." Ph.D. dissertation, University of California, Berkeley.

————. 1993a. "The shaman's destiny: Symptoms, affliction, and the re-interpretation of illness among the Taman." In *The Seen and the Unseen: Shamanism, Mediumship and Possession in Borneo,* edited by Robert L. Winzeler, pp. 171–206. Monograph Series of the Borneo Research Council, vol. 2. Williamsburg, VA: Borneo Research Council.

————. 1993b. "Poisons and antidotes among the Taman of West Kalimantan, Indonesia." *Bijdragen tot de Taal-, Land- en Volkenkunde* 149: 3–21.

————. 1994. "*Kempunan*: An Indigenous Explanation of Misfortune and Illness in Borneo and Peninsular Malaysia." Paper presented at the 93rd annual meeting of the American Anthropological Association, Atlanta, GA.

————. n.d. "Spirit Attack and Soul Capture: The Explanation and Treatment of Serious Illness Among the Taman." Unpublished manuscript.

Blacker, Kay, and Joe P. Tupin. 1977. "Hysteria and hysterical structures: Developmental and social theories." In *Hysterical Personality,* edited by Mardi J. Horowitz, pp. 97–141. New York: Jason Aronson.

Bourguignon, Erika. 1965. "The self, the behavioral environment, and the theory of spirit possession." In *Context and Meaning in Cultural Anthropology,* edited by Melford E. Spiro, pp. 39–60. New York: The Free Press.

Boyer, Pascal. 1993. "Pseudo-natural kinds." In *Cognitive Aspects of Religious Symbolism,* edited by Pascal Boyer, pp. 121–141. Cambridge: Cambridge University Press.

Brown, Cecil H. 1984. *Language and Living Things: Uniformities in Folk-Classification and Naming.* New Brunswick, NJ: Rutgers University Press.

Brown, Donald E. 1991. "The penis pin: an unsolved problem in the relations between the sexes in Borneo." In *Female and Male in Borneo: Contributions and Challenges to Gender Studies,* edited by Vinson H. Sutlive, Jr., pp. 435–454. Borneo Research Council Monograph Series, vol. 1. Williamsburg, VA: Borneo Research Council.

Brown, Donald E., James W. Edwards, and Ruth Moore. 1988. *The Penis Inserts of Southeast Asia: An Annotated Bibliography with an Overview and Comparative Perspectives.* Occasional Paper no. 15. Berkeley: Center for South and Southeast Asian Studies, University of California, Berkeley.

Carneiro, Robert L. 1973. "The four faces of evolution." In *Handbook of Social and Cultural Anthropology,* edited by John J. Honigmann, pp. 89–110. Chicago: Rand McNally and Company.

Chu, Clayton H. 1978. "The Three Worlds of Iban Shamanism." Ph.D. dissertation, Columbia University.

Crocker, Jon Christopher. 1985. *Vital Souls: Bororo Cosmology, Natural Symbolism, and Shamanism.* Tucson: University of Arizona Press.

Csordas, Thomas J. 1993. "Somatic modes of attention." *Cultural Anthropology* 8: 135–156.

Dalton, George. 1967. "Primitive money." In *Tribal and Peasant Economies: Readings in Economic Anthropology,* edited by George Dalton, pp. 254–281. Garden City, NY: Natural History Press.

Deutsch, Helene. 1944–1945. *The Psychology of Women.* 2 vols. New York: Grune & Stratton.

Devereux, George. 1980. "Normal and abnormal." In *Basic Problems of Ethnopsychiatry,* translated by Basia Miller Gulati and George Devereux, pp. 3–71. Chicago: University of Chicago Press.

De Vos, George A. 1974. "Cross-cultural studies of mental disorder: An anthropological perspective." In *American Handbook of Psychiatry,* edited by Gerald Caplan, vol. 3, pp. 551–567. New York: Basic Books.

————. 1980. "Psychological anthropology: Humans as learners of culture." In *People in Culture,* edited by Ino Rossi, pp. 170–224. New York: Praeger.

————. 1983. "Adaptive conflict and adjustive coping: Psychocultural approaches to ethnic identity." In *Studies in Social Identity,* edited by T. Sarbin and K. Scheibe, pp. 204–230. New York: Praeger.

————. 1990. *Status Inequality: A Psychocultural Approach to the Self.* Newbury Park, CA: Sage.

Dharma, A. P. 1985. *Tanaman Obat Tradisional Indonesia (Medicinal Plants in Indonesian Traditional Medicine).* Jakarta: PN Balai Pustaka.

Diposiswoyo, Mudiyono. 1985. "Tradition et changement social: Etude ethnographique des Taman de Kalimantan Ouest" ("Tradition and Social Change: An Ethnographic Study of the Taman of Kalimantan"). Thèse de doctorat de 3ème cycle, Ecole des Hautes Etudes en Sciences Sociales.

Dolgin, Janet L., David M. Kemnitzer, and David M. Schneider, editors. 1977. *Symbolic Anthropology: A Reader in the Study of Symbols and Meanings.* New York: Columbia University Press.

Durkheim, Emile. 1976 [1912]. *The Elementary Forms of Religious Life,* translated by Joseph Swain. Second edition. London: George Allen and Unwin.

Echols, John M., and Hassan Shadily. 1989. *An Indonesian-English Dictionary.* Third edition, revised and edited by John U. Wolff, James T. Collins, and Hassan Shadily. Ithaca, NY: Cornell University Press.

Eisenberg, Leon. 1977. "Disease and illness: Distinctions between professional and popular ideas of sickness." *Culture, Medicine, and Psychiatry* 1: 9–23.

Eliade, Mircea. 1964 [1951]. *Shamanism: Archaic Techniques of Ecstasy,* translated by Willard R. Trask. Bollingen Series, no. 76. Princeton, NJ: Princeton University Press.

Elkin, A. P. 1977. *Aboriginal Men of High Degree.* Second edition. New York: St. Martin's Press.

Endicott, Kirk Michael. 1970. *An Analysis of Malay Magic.* Oxford: Clarendon Press.

Epstein, Cynthia Fuchs. 1970. *Women's Place: Options and Limits in Professional Careers.* Berkeley: University of California Press.

Etkin, Nina L. 1988. "Cultural constructions of efficacy." In *The Context of Medicines in Developing Countries,* edited by S. van der Geest and S. R. White, pp. 299–326. Dordrecht, Netherlands: Kluwer Academic Publishers.

Fenichel, Otto. 1945. *The Psychoanalytic Theory of Neurosis.* New York: W. W. Norton.

Firth, Raymond. 1967. *Tikopia Ritual and Belief.* Boston: Beacon Press.

————. 1973. *Symbols: Public and Private.* Ithaca, NY: Cornell University Press.

Flaherty, Gloria. 1992. *Shamanism and the Eighteenth Century.* Princeton, NJ: Princeton University Press.

Foster, George M. 1976. "Disease etiologies in non-Western medical systems." *American Anthropologist* 78: 773–782.

Frankenberg, Ronald. 1980. "Medical anthropology and development: a theoretical perspective." *Social Science and Medicine* 14B: 197–207.

Freeman, Derek. 1958. "The family system of the Iban of Borneo." In *The Developmental Cycle in Domestic Groups,* edited by Jack Goody, pp. 15–52. Cambridge Papers in Social Anthropology, no. 1. Cambridge: Cambridge University Press.

———. 1967. "Shaman and incubus." *Psychoanalytic Study of Society* 4: 315–343.

———. 1970. *Report on the Iban.* London School of Economics Monographs on Social Anthropology, no. 41. London: Athlone Press.

Freidson, Eliot. 1970. *Profession of Medicine: A Study of the Sociology of Applied Knowledge.* New York: Dodd, Mead & Co.

Gadow, Sally. 1982. "Body and self: A dialectic." In *The Humanity of the Ill: Phenomenological Perspectives,* edited by Victor Kestenbaum, pp. 142–156. Knoxville: University of Tennessee Press.

Gell, Alfred. 1974. "Understanding the occult." *Radical Philosophy* 9: 17–26.

———. 1980. "The gods at play: vertigo and possession in Muria religion." *Man* 15: 219–248.

Gimlette, John D. 1971 [1929]. *Malay Poisons and Charm Cures.* Reprint of third edition. Singapore: Oxford University Press.

Golomb, Louis. 1985. *An Anthropology of Curing in Multiethnic Thailand.* Urbana: University of Illinois Press.

Good, Byron J. 1994. *Medicine, Rationality, and Experience: An Anthropological Perspective.* Cambridge: Cambridge University Press.

Goode, William J. 1951. *Religion Among the Primitives.* New York: The Free Press.

Goodman, Felicitas D. 1990. *Where the Spirits Ride the Wind: Trance Journeys and Other Ecstatic Experiences.* Bloomington: Indiana University Press.

Graham, Penelope. 1987. *Iban Shamanism: An Analysis of the Ethnographic Literature.* An occasional paper of the Department of Anthropology. Canberra: Research School of Pacific Studies, Australian National University.

Gregory, James R. 1984. "The myth of the male ethnographer and the women's world." *American Anthropologist* 86: 313–327.

Grim, John A. 1983. *The Shaman: Patterns of Religious Healing Among the Ojibway Indians.* Norman: University of Oklahoma Press.

Harner, Michael J. 1973. "The sound of rushing water." In *Hallucinogens and Shamanism,* edited by Michael J. Harner, pp. 15–27. London: Oxford University Press.

———. 1980. *The Way of the Shaman: A Guide to Power and Healing.* New York: Bantam Books.

Harrisson, Tom. 1962. "Borneo death." *Bijdragen tot de Taal-, Land- en Volkenkunde* 118: 1–41.

———. 1965. "The Malohs of Kalimantan: Ethnological notes." *Sarawak Museum Journal* 12: 236–350.

———. 1966. "Maloh coffin designs." *Sarawak Museum Journal* 14: 146–150.

Helms, Mary W. 1988. *Ulysses' Sail: An Ethnographic Odyssey of Power, Knowledge, and Geographical Distance.* Princeton, NJ: Princeton University Press.

Hose, Charles, and William McDougall. 1912. *The Pagan Tribes of Borneo.* 2 vols. London: Macmillan.

Hudson, A. B. 1970. "A note on Selako: Malayic Dayak and Land Dayak languages in Western Borneo." *Sarawak Museum Journal* 18: 301–318.

―――. 1978. "Linguistic relations among Bornean peoples with special reference to Sarawak: An interim report." *Studies in Third World Societies* (Publication 3: "Sarawak: Linguistics and Development Problems"): 1–44.

Hultkrantz, Åke. 1978. "Ecological and phenomenological aspects of shamanism." In *Shamanism in Siberia,* edited by V. Diószegi and M. Hoppál, pp. 27–58. Bibliotheca Uralica 1. Budapest: Akadémiai Kiadó.

Jacobus E. Frans L., S. 1992. "The customary death ceremony of the Dayak Banuaka' community in Kapuas Hulu Regency, Kalimantan Barat Province." Paper presented at the Borneo Research Council Second Biennial International Conference, Kota Kinabalu.

Jamuh, George. 1960. "Ideas about poisoning." *Sarawak Museum Journal* 9: 461–467.

Jules-Rosette, Benetta. 1975. "Song and spirit: The use of songs in the management of ritual contexts." *Africa* 45: 150–166.

Kapferer, Bruce. 1977. "First class to Maradana: Secular drama in Sinhalese healing rites." In *Secular Ritual,* edited by Sally F. Moore and Barbara G. Myerhoff, pp. 91–123. Assen, Neth.: Van Gorcum.

―――. 1991. *A Celebration of Demons: Exorcism and the Aesthetics of Healing in Sri Lanka.* Second edition. Providence, RI: Berghahn.

Keeler, Ward. 1987. *Javanese Shadow Plays, Javanese Selves.* Princeton, NJ: Princeton University Press.

Keesing, Roger M. 1987. "Anthropology as interpretive quest." *Current Anthropology* 28: 161–176.

Kennedy, John G. 1973. "Cultural psychiatry." In *Handbook of Social and Cultural Anthropology,* edited by John J. Honigmann, pp. 1119–1198. Chicago: Rand McNally and Co.

Kimball, Linda Amy. 1979. *Borneo Medicine: The Healing Art of Indigenous Brunei Malay Medicine.* Ann Arbor, MI: University Microfilms International.

King, Victor T. 1975. "Stones and the Maloh of Indonesian West Borneo." *Journal of the Malaysian Branch of the Royal Asiatic Society* 48(1): 104–119.

―――. 1976a. "Cursing, special death and spirits in Embaloh society." *Bijdragen tot de Taal-, Land- en Volkenkunde* 132: 124–145.

―――. 1976b. "The Maloh language: A vocabulary and summary of the literature." *Sarawak Museum Journal* 24: 137–164.

―――. 1985. *The Maloh of West Kalimantan: An Ethnographic Study of Social Inequality and Social Change Among an Indonesian Borneo People.* Verhandelingen van het Koninklijk Instituut voor Taal-, Land- en Volkenkunde, no.108. Dordrecht, Netherlands: Foris Publications.

―――. 1993. *The Peoples of Borneo.* Oxford: Blackwell.

Kleinman, Arthur. 1978. "Concepts and a model for the comparison of medical systems as cultural systems." *Social Science and Medicine* 12B: 85–93.

―――. 1988. *The Illness Narratives: Suffering, Healing, and the Human Condition.* New York: Basic Books.

Krohn, Alan. 1978. *Hysteria: The Elusive Neurosis.* Psychological Issues 12:1/2 Monograph 45/46. New York: International Universities Press.

La Barre, Weston. 1972. *The Ghost Dance: Origins of Religion.* New York: Dell Publishing Co.

Laderman, Carol. 1991. *Taming the Wind of Desire: Psychology, Medicine, and Aesthetics in Malay Shamanistic Performance.* Berkeley: University of

California Press.

Leitenberg, Harold, and Kris Henning. 1995. "Sexual fantasy." *Psychological Bulletin* 117: 469–496.

Levinson, Daniel J. 1978. *The Seasons of a Man's Life.* New York: Alfred A. Knopf.

Lévi-Strauss, Claude. 1963 [1958]. *Structural Anthropology,* translated by Claire Jacobson and Brooke Grundfest Schoepf. New York: Basic Books.

————. 1966 [1962]. *The Savage Mind.* Chicago: University of Chicago Press.

Lewis, I. M. 1971. *Ecstatic Religion: An Anthropological Study of Spirit Possession and Shamanism.* Harmondsworth, England: Penguin.

————. 1986. *Religion in Context: Cults and Charisma.* Cambridge: Cambridge University Press.

Luhrmann, T. M. 1989. *Persuasions of the Witch's Craft: Ritual Magic in Contemporary England.* Cambridge: Harvard University Press.

Macdonald, D. B., and H. Massé. 1965. "Djinn." In *The Encyclopedia of Islam,* new edition, vol. 2, pp. 546–550. Leiden, Netherlands: E. J. Brill.

Marcus, George E., and Michael M. J. Fischer. 1986. *Anthropology as Cultural Critique: An Experimental Moment in the Human Sciences.* Chicago: University of Chicago Press.

Meadows, Kenneth. 1991. *Shamanic Experience: A Practical Guide to Contemporary Shamanism.* Shaftesbury, England: Element.

Metcalf, Peter. 1982. *A Borneo Journey into Death: Berawan Eschatology Through Its Rituals.* Philadelphia: University of Pennsylvania Press.

Mohd. Taib bin Osman. 1972. "Patterns of supernatural premises underlying the institution of the *bomoh* in Malay culture." *Bijdragen tot de Taal-, Land- en Volkenkunde* 128: 219–234.

Morinis, Alan. 1985. "The ritual experience: Pain and the transformation of consciousness in ordeals of initiation." *Ethos* 13: 150–174.

Mujarrobat Madiinatul Asroor. 1980? 2 vols. Jakarta: M.A. Jaya.

Murray, Stephen O. 1992. "Late-nineteenth century reports on manangs in northern Borneo." In *Oceanic Homosexualities,* edited by Stephen O. Murray, pp. 285–292. Garland Gay and Lesbian Series, no. 7. New York: Garland Publishing, Inc.

Needham, Rodney. 1967. "Blood, thunder, and the mockery of animals." In *Myth and Cosmos: Readings in Mythology and Symbolism,* edited by John Middleton, pp. 271–285. Garden City, NY: The Natural History Press.

————. 1979. "Percussion and transition." In *Reader in Comparative Religion: An Anthropological Approach,* edited by William A. Lessa and Evon Z. Vogt, fourth edition, pp. 311–318. New York: Harper and Row.

Neher, Andrew. 1962. "A physiological explanation of unusual behavior in ceremonies involving drums." *Human Biology* 34: 151–160.

————. 1990. *The Psychology of Transcendence.* Second edition. New York: Dover Publications, Inc.

Nemiah, John C. 1988. "Psychoneurotic disorders." In *The New Harvard Guide to Psychiatry,* edited by Armand M. Nicholi, Jr., pp. 234–258. Cambridge: Harvard University Press.

Obeyesekere, Gananath. 1981. *Medusa's Hair: An Essay on Personal Symbols and Religious Experience.* Chicago: The University of Chicago Press.

Parsons, Anne. 1969. *Belief, Magic, and Anomie: Essays in Psychosocial Anthropology.* New York: The Free Press.

Payne, Kenneth William. 1985. "The Sulphur Eaters: Illness, Its Ritual, and the Social Order Among the Tagabawa Bagobos of Southcentral Mindanao, Philippines." Ph.D. dissertation, University of California, Berkeley.

Pellegrino, Edmund D., and David C. Thomasma. 1981. *A Philosophical Basis of*

Medical Practice: Toward a Philosophy and Ethic of the Healing Professions. New York: Oxford University Press.

Price-Williams, Douglass. 1987. "The waking dream in ethnographic perspective." In *Dreaming: Anthropological and Psychological Interpretations,* pp. 246–262. Cambridge: Cambridge University Press.

Rabinow, Paul, and William M. Sullivan, editors. 1979. *Interpretive Social Science: A Reader.* Berkeley: University of California Press.

Rancour-Laferriere, Daniel. 1985. *Signs of the Flesh: An Essay on the Evolution of Hominid Sexuality.* Bloomington: Indiana University Press.

Rank, Otto. 1971 [1922]. *The Double: A Psychoanalytic Study,* translated, edited, and with an introduction by Harry Tucker, Jr. Chapel Hill: University of North Carolina Press.

Riches, David. 1994. "Shamanism: The key to religion." *Man* 29: 381–405.

Róheim, Géza. 1930. *Animism, Magic, and the Divine King.* New York: Alfred A. Knopf.

———. 1952. *The Gates of the Dream.* New York: International Universities Press.

Rouget, Gilbert. 1980. *Music and Trance.* Chicago: University of Chicago Press.

Rousseau, Jérôme. 1990. *Central Borneo: Ethnic Identity and Social Life in a Stratified Society.* Oxford: Clarendon Press.

Sastrowardoyo, Pandil, M. Kasim Thaha, Suhamie Zahra, Mas Irawan Sugiran, and M. Ikot Rinding. 1983/1984. *Upacara Tradisional Yang Berkaitan Dengan Peristiwa Alam Dan Kepercayaan Daerah Kalimantan Barat (Traditional Ceremonies Associated with Natural Events and Beliefs in the West Kalimantan Region).* Pontianak?: Departemen Pendidikan dan Kebudayaan.

Sather, Clifford. 1978. "The malevolent *koklir*: Iban concepts of sexual peril and the dangers of childbirth." *Bijdragen tot de Taal-, Land- en Volkenkunde* 134: 310–355.

———. 1993. "Shaman and fool: Representations of the shaman in Iban comic fables." In *The Seen and the Unseen: Shamanism, Mediumship and Possession in Borneo,* edited by Robert L. Winzeler, pp. 281–322. Borneo Research Council Monograph Series, vol. 2. Williamsburg, VA: Borneo Research Council.

———. 1994. "The one-sided one: Iban rice myths, agricultural ritual and notions of ancestors." *Contributions to Southeast Asian Ethnography* 10: 119–150.

Scheper-Hughes, Nancy. 1994. "Embodied knowledge: Thinking with the body in critical medical anthropology." In *Assessing Cultural Anthropology,* edited by Robert Borofsky, pp. 229–239. New York: McGraw-Hill.

Schieffelin, Edward L. 1985. "Performance and the cultural construction of reality." *American Ethnologist* 12: 707–724.

Schwartz, Theodore. 1976. "The cargo cult: A Melanesian type-response to change." In *Responses to Change: Society, Culture, and Personality,* edited by George A. De Vos, pp. 157–206. New York: D. Van Nostrand Reinhold Co.

Shapiro, David. 1965. *Neurotic Styles.* New York: Basic Books.

Sharp, Lesley Alexandra. 1990. "The Possessed and the Dispossessed: Spirits, Identity, and Power in a Madagascar Migrant Town." Ph.D. dissertation, University of California, Berkeley.

Shorter, Edward. 1992. *From Paralysis to Fatigue: A History of Psychosomatic Illness in the Modern Era.* New York: The Free Press.

———. 1994. *From the Body into the Mind: The Cultural Origins of Psychosomatic Symptoms.* New York: The Free Press.

Siikala, Anna-Leena. 1978. *The Rite Technique of the Siberian Shaman.* FF Communications, no. 220. Helsinki: Suomalainen Tiedeakatemia.

Siong, Bartholomeus Moses. 1984. "Beberapa Faktor Sosial Budaya Yang Ikut

Berperan Dalam Terjadinya Perceraian Dikalangan Suku Dayak Taman Kristen Di Sibau Hilir" ("Some Sociocultural Factors Affecting the Occurrence of Divorce Among the Christian Taman Dayaks in Sibau Hilir"). Tesis Sarjana, Fakultas Theologia, Universitas Kristen Satya Wacana.

Skeat, Walter William. 1900. *Malay Magic: An Introduction to the Folklore and Popular Religion of the Malay Peninsular.* London: Macmillan.

Slaats, Herman, and Karen Portier. 1993. "Sorcery and the law in modern Indonesia." In *Understanding Witchcraft and Sorcery in Southeast Asia,* edited by C. W. Watson and Roy Ellen, pp. 135–148. Honolulu: University of Hawaii Press.

Slater, Candace. 1994. *Dance of the Dolphin: Transformation and Disenchantment in the Amazonian Imagination.* Chicago: The University of Chicago Press.

Sungkalang, Silvanus. 1982. "Proses Penyelesaian Perkara Menurut Hukum Adat Pada Suku Daya Taman Di Kecamatan Putussibau Kabupaten Kapuas Hulu" ("The Conflict Resolution Process in the Customary Law of the Taman Dayaks of Putussibau Subdistrict, Upper Kapuas Regency"). Skripsi Sarjana, Fakultas Hukum, Universitas Tanjungpura.

Sutlive, Vinson H., Jr. 1992. "The Iban manang in the Sibu district of the Third Division of Sarawak: An alternate route to normality." In *Oceanic Homosexualities,* edited by Stephen O. Murray, pp. 273–284. Garland Gay and Lesbian Series, no. 7. New York: Garland Publishing, Inc.

Sweeney, Amin. 1987. *A Full Hearing: Orality and Literacy in the Malay World.* Berkeley: University of California Press.

Tambiah, Stanley Jeyaraja. 1985. *Culture, Thought, and Social Action: An Anthropological Perspective.* Cambridge: Harvard University Press.

Tampubolon, Oswald T. 1981. *Tumbuhan Obat: Bagi Pencinta Alam (Medicinal Plants: For Nature Lovers).* Jakarta: Penerbit Bhratara Aksara.

Tsing, Anna Lowenhaupt. 1987. "A rhetoric of centers in a religion of the periphery." In *Indonesian Religions in Transition,* edited by Rita S. Kipp and Susan Rodgers, pp. 187–210. Tucson: University of Arizona Press.

———. 1993. *In the Realm of the Diamond Queen: Marginality in an Out-of-the-Way Place.* Princeton, NJ: Princeton University Press.

Turner, Terence S. 1977. "Transformation, hierarchy and transcendence: A reformulation of Van Gennep's model of the structure of rites de passage." In *Secular Ritual,* edited by Sally F. Moore and Barbara G. Myerhoff, pp. 53–70. Assen, Netherlands: Van Gorcum.

Turner, Victor W. 1967. *The Forest of Symbols: Aspects of Ndembu Ritual.* Ithaca, NY: Cornell University Press.

———. 1968. *The Drums of Affliction: A Study of Religious Processes Among the Ndembu of Zambia.* Oxford: Clarendon Press.

———. 1969. *The Ritual Process: Structure and Anti-structure.* Chicago: Aldine.

———. 1974. *Dramas, Fields, and Metaphors: Symbolic Action in Human Societies.* Ithaca, NY: Cornell University Press.

Valory, Dale Keith. 1970. "Yurok Doctors and Devils: A Study in Identity, Anxiety and Deviance." Ph.D. dissertation, University of California, Berkeley.

Van Gennep, Arnold. 1960 [1909]. *The Rites of Passage,* translated by M. B. Vizedom and G. L. Caffee. Chicago: University of Chicago Press.

Walsh, Roger N. 1990. *The Spirit of Shamanism.* Los Angeles: Jeremy P. Tarcher, Inc.

Watson, C. W. 1987. *State and Society in Indonesia.* Occasional Paper no. 8. Canterbury: Centre of South-East Asian Studies, University of Kent at Canterbury.

Weber, Max. 1964 [1947]. *The Theory of Social and Economic Organization,* translated by A. M. Henderson and T. Parsons. New York: The Free Press.

Weiner, Annette B. 1992. *Inalienable Possessions: The Paradox of Keeping-While-Giving.* Berkeley: University of California Press.

———. 1994. "Cultural difference and the density of objects." (AES distinguished lecture.) *American Ethnologist* 21: 391–403.

Weinstock, Joseph A. 1987. "Kaharingan: Life and death in southern Borneo." In *Indonesian Religions in Transition,* edited by Rita Smith Kipp and Susan Rodgers, pp. 71–97. Tucson: University of Arizona Press.

Whittier, Herbert Lincoln. 1973. "Social Organization and Symbols of Social Differentiation: An Ethnographic Study of the Kenyah Dayak of East Kalimantan (Borneo)." Ph.D. dissertation, Michigan State University.

Wikan, Unni. 1990. *Managing Turbulent Hearts: A Balinese Formula for Living.* Chicago: University of Chicago Press.

Wilkinson, R. J. 1901. *A Malay-English Dictionary.* Singapore: Kelly and Walsh.

Wilson, Bryan R. 1973. *Magic and the Millennium: A Sociological Study of Religious Movements of Protest Among Tribal and Third-World Peoples.* London: Heinemann.

Winkelman, Michael James. 1992. *Shamans, Priests and Witches: A Cross-Cultural Study of Magico-Religious Practitioners.* Anthropological Research Papers no. 44. Tempe: Arizona State University.

Winkler, John J. 1990. *The Constraints of Desire: The Anthropology of Sex and Gender in Ancient Greece.* New York: Routledge.

Winstedt, Richard. 1951. *The Malay Magician, Being Shaman, Saiva and Sufi.* London: Routledge and Kegan Paul.

Winzeler, Robert L. 1993. "Shaman, priest, and spirit medium: Religious specialists, tradition and innovation in Borneo." In *The Seen and the Unseen: Shamanism, Mediumship and Possession in Borneo,* edited by Robert L. Winzeler, pp. xi–xxxiii. Borneo Research Council Monograph Series, vol. 2. Williamsburg, VA: Borneo Research Council.

———, editor. 1993. *The Seen and the Unseen: Shamanism, Mediumship and Possession in Borneo.* Borneo Research Council Monograph Series, vol. 2. Williamsburg, VA: Borneo Research Council.

Yates, Frances A. 1966. *The Art of Memory.* Chicago: University of Chicago Press.

Young, Allan. 1975. "Magic as a 'quasi-profession': The organization of magic and magical healers among Amhara." *Ethnology* 14: 245–265.

———. 1976a. "Some implications of medical beliefs and practices for social anthropology." *American Anthropologist* 78: 5–25.

———. 1976b. "Internalizing and externalizing medical belief systems: An Ethiopian example." *Social Science and Medicine* 10: 147–156.

Index

Adultery, 21, 25, 40
Agama Jolo, 26–27
Agriculture, 28–30, 135–136. *See also*
Shifting cultivation
Alatala, 26, 30*n7*
Ali (dukun), 44, 48
Amulets, 41, 42, 44, 48
Animals, used in ceremonies, 98
Animism, 26, 28, 117
Antidotes, 34, 36–38, 43, 106*n8*
Antu. *See* Ghosts
Anxiety, 9, 79
Areca catechu, 105. *See also* Mayang
pinang
Astrology, 42
Atkinson, Jane, 3–5, 8, 160–161
Augury, areca blossom, 98–99, 99*il*,
133, 145
Authority, political, 4

Badi, 65–67, 74*n9*, 82
Balienism, 161*n7;* advancement in,
157–158; as career, 156–158; changing meanings in, 163–171; concepts
of souls, 57–65; concepts of spirits,
54–57; customary practice in, 146;
deception in, 10, 11, 160; efficacy
of, 158–161; in ethnomedical
domain, 6; gender in, 4, 5, 12,
106*n6*, 145, 151–154, 167–168;
hierarchy of, 143; institutionalization of, 141; knowledge in, 6–7;
legitimacy of, 143, 146; as magic,
142–144; mystification in, 11;
objects used, 133–136; as organized

activity, 141–147; predisposing conditions, 77–86; as profession,
141–149; psychological perspective,
8; resistance to, 85–86; sexual
repression in, 9, 83, 170; simplifica-
tion of, 166; social organization of,
145–147; social pressure in, 85–86;
social reality of, 158–161; in society, 141–161; support from kin in,
155–156
Baliens, 74; apprenticeship, 124;
authenticity of, 104; becoming,
77–105, 150–156; celestial, 149;
commitment of, 105; compensation
for, 31, 38, 39, 99–100, 133–134,
136, 139*n11;* deceased, 125, 147,
149; destiny of, 84–85; equipment
for, 89, 95, 101, 109–138, 116,
118–119, 133; esotericism of,
149–150; identity, 7; illness in,
150–151, 156; inauguration of, 1;
for initiation ceremony, 87; involuntary nature of, 2, 77; kinship choice,
117; obligations of, 112, 156; psychological health of, 5, 154–155;
ranking, 148–149; recruitment of, 8;
role change of, 11; sarin, 149; selection for bubut, 114–115; selection
for mangait, 117–118; status of, 5, 7,
147–150, 167; techniques of,
109–138; terrestrial, 149
Banuakas, 18–19, 20, 23
Baudrilliard, Jean, 134–135
Belief(s): cultural, 144; customary, 26;
effects on pain, 104; kempunan, 35,

About the Book

This fascinating case study focuses on shamanism and the healing practices of the Taman, a formerly tribal society indigenous to the interior of Borneo. The Taman typically associate illness with an encounter with spirits that both seduce and torment a person in dreams or waking life. Rather than use medicines to counter the effect of these discomforting visitors, the shamans—called baliens—use stones that are thought to have come into being by materializing wild spirits that have converged during the initiation ceremony.

Jay Bernstein argues that shamanism continues to flourish not merely because of tradition, but because it meets real needs for therapy that are not otherwise satisfied. He stresses the exchange of objects in shamanic ceremonies and argues for the relevance of psychology and symbolic and social processes in explaining the identity of shamans. Finally, he situates Taman shamanism in the context of the pluralistic medical system of interior Borneo, which includes the traditions of the nearby Malay Muslims and Iban Dayaks.

Written in a style that will engage the interest of both scholars and beginning students, *Spirits Captured in Stone* is a valuable contribution to contemporary debates in cultural and medical anthropology; the anthropology of religion, as well as magic and ritual; folklore; and Southeast Asian ethnography.

Jay H. Bernstein is a research affiliate in the Division of Library and Information Science and the University Library, St. John's University.